THE YEAR-ROUND ANTI-INFLAMMATORY DIET COOKBOOK FOR BEGINNERS

2000 Days of Delicious and Nutritious Recipes, a 60-Day Meal Plan, and 3 Bonus to Reduce Inflammation, Enhance Immunity, and Boost Health

Patricia Harper

Table of Contents

INTRODUCTION

Welcome to the world of anti-inflammatory cooking

Welcome to the world of anti-inflammatory cooking! In this culinary journey, we will take you through a tasty and healthy journey, where flavors combine with wellness to create delicious and nutritious dishes.

Anti-inflammatory cooking is more than just a diet; it is a lifestyle that promotes better health and well-being. This cuisine is designed to help your body fight inflammation naturally by providing nutrition and beneficial substances through carefully selected ingredients.

You can expect a wide range of colorful and appetizing dishes, including ingredients such as fresh fruits, crunchy vegetables, lean proteins, herbs, and exotic spices. We will not only delight you with tasty recipes, but also help you understand the link between nutrition and health by providing clear and accessible information.

This guide is designed for those new to anti-inflammatory cooking. You do not need to be an experienced chef or nutritionist to appreciate the benefits of this cuisine. We have made everything simple and understandable so that you can begin this journey without any complications.

We are here to be your fellow travelers, providing you with tips, advice and practical recipes to make your approach to anti-inflammatory cooking easy and fun. Each step you take toward an anti-inflammatory diet will bring you closer to a healthier life in harmony with your body.

So, get ready to discover a new world of flavors, explore exotic ingredients, and experience the wellness that anti-inflammatory cooking can bring to your life. Are you ready to begin this culinary adventure with us? Buckle up and get ready to enjoy anti-inflammatory cooking!

Understanding Inflammation and the Importance of Diet for Health

Inflammation is our body's natural reaction to injury, infection, or irritation. When the immune system senses a potential threat, it triggers a defense mechanism to protect and heal damaged tissues. Although it is an essential process for healing, chronic inflammation can have a negative impact on our health and can be associated with several pathological conditions.

Inflammation and General Health

Understanding the concept of inflammation is critical to appreciating how diet can play a crucial role in our overall health. Chronic inflammation, though less obvious than acute symptoms, can be a silent force that threatens our long-term well-being.

Persistent inflammation in our bodies can damage cells and tissues, contributing to chronic diseases such as heart disease, type 2 diabetes, rheumatoid arthritis, asthma, obesity, and even some forms of cancer. In addition, chronic inflammation has been linked to mood disorders and mental conditions such as depression and anxiety.

The Key Role of Diet

The good news is that we can influence the level of inflammation in our bodies through conscious food choices. Anti-inflammatory cooking is based on foods that have been shown to have anti-inflammatory properties and abilities to support our immune system.

Some of the anti-inflammatory heroes found in the anti-inflammatory kitchen include dark green leafy vegetables such as spinach and kale, which are rich in antioxidants and vitamins. Berries, such as blueberries and strawberries, are full of beneficial phytochemical compounds. Nuts and seeds provide omega-3 fatty acids and polyphenols, helping to reduce inflammation.

Extra-virgin olive oil and fatty fish, such as salmon and sardines, are valuable sources of healthy fats that have been shown to have positive effects on heart health and reduced inflammation. And, of course, aromatic spices such as turmeric, ginger, cinnamon, and black pepper, to name a few, can give our dishes extraordinary flavor and enhance the anti-inflammatory properties of our meals.

A Healthy and Tasty Kitchen

Our anti-inflammatory cooking is not only about health, but also about pleasure and taste. You don't have to worry about giving up flavor or meal satisfaction. You will discover how to combine nutritious ingredients in creative ways to create delicious dishes that not only nourish your body, but also your spirit.

In this guide, we will teach you to explore your culinary side and embrace a cuisine that offers nourishment and gratification, without ever sacrificing the pleasure of food. You will discover how even everyday dishes can be transformed into enjoyable and nourishing culinary experiences, enriching your well-being in every bite.

A Healthier and Vibrant Life

Understanding the link between inflammation and diet offers us the opportunity to take our health and well-being into our own hands. Anti-inflammatory cooking is an invitation to a healthier, more vibrant life, where food choices become acts of love toward our bodies and minds.

Get ready to explore a world of flavor, discovery, and health as we take you on this culinary journey to anti-inflammatory cooking. We are excited to share with you tasty recipes, practical tips and knowledge to help you embark on this culinary adventure toward a healthier and happier future.

CHAPTER 1
How the process of inflammation works: the importance of diet

1: The Role of Inflammation in the Body.

Inflammation is our body's natural reaction to injury, infection, or irritation. When the immune system senses a potential threat, it triggers a defense mechanism to protect and heal damaged tissues. This protective mechanism is essential to the healing process and to keeping our bodies safe from potential threats.

During the process of inflammation, our body precisely coordinates a series of reactions to deal with the ongoing threat:

- o Activation of immune system cells: Leukocytes, the white blood cells of our immune system, detect the presence of harmful agents and are activated to fight them.
- o Dilation of blood vessels: Blood vessels in the affected area dilate, increasing blood flow to that specific area, causing redness and warming of the area.
- o Increased vascular permeability: Blood vessels become more permeable, allowing immune cells and fluids to escape from the vessels and reach the affected tissue, contributing to edema and swelling.
- o Influx of immune cells: Immune cells, such as leukocytes, crowd the inflamed area, ready to attack and neutralize invading pathogens or repair damaged tissue.
- o Production of cytokines and prostaglandins: During the inflammatory process, our body produces special chemicals called cytokines and prostaglandins that regulate inflammation and pain.
- o Communication of chemicals: Cytokines and prostaglandins communicate with cells of the immune system, coordinating the inflammatory response and the beginning of the resolution phase, in which inflammation gradually decreases and our body begins the process of tissue healing and repair.

Inflammation is a vital mechanism for our well-being, but when it becomes chronic it can damage healthy cells and cause health problems. Chronic inflammation has been linked to several chronic diseases, such as heart disease, type 2 diabetes, arthritis, autoimmune diseases, and gastrointestinal disorders. In addition, scientific studies have highlighted the key role of inflammation in cellular aging and cognitive impairment.

Fortunately, we can influence inflammation in our bodies through conscious food choices. A diet rich in anti-inflammatory foods can help reduce inflammation and promote optimal health. In the next few subchapters, we will explore the best anti-inflammatory foods that we should include in our diet to promote well-being and overall health. You will discover how to combine these ingredients in creative and delicious ways to create dishes that are a feast for the senses and a balm for the body.

Anti-inflammatory cooking is an opportunity to embrace a new culinary lifestyle in which a love of food is combined with care for our bodies. Get ready to discover a world of flavors and benefits as we delve into the magical universe of anti-inflammatory cooking!

2: How Diet Can Affect Inflammation.

We have seen how inflammation is a natural and necessary process for our health, but also how chronic inflammation can have a negative impact on our well-being. Now you may be wondering, "How can we influence inflammation through our diet?" Well, you have raised a fundamental question!

Diet plays a crucial role in regulating inflammation in our bodies. There are foods that can trigger an inflammatory response in our bodies, while others have anti-inflammatory properties, helping to reduce inflammation and promote better health.

Avoiding Pro-Inflammatory Foods

Foods high in added sugars, saturated fats and refined vegetable oils can be considered pro-inflammatory. These include foods such as:

Sweets and sugary drinks: sweets, carbonated drinks and sugary snacks can trigger an inflammatory response in our body.

Fatty meats and whole dairy products: foods high in saturated fats, such as nonfat red meats and whole dairy products, can increase inflammation levels.

Refined vegetable oils: oils such as corn, soybean, and sunflower oil may contain excess omega-6 fatty acids, which can contribute to inflammation if consumed in large quantities.

Embracing Anti-Inflammatory Foods

Fortunately, there is a world of foods with anti-inflammatory properties that can help us fight inflammation and improve our health. Here are some of them:

Berries: blueberries, raspberries and strawberries are rich in antioxidants and anti-inflammatory compounds.

Green leafy vegetables: spinach, kale, arugula and other green leafy vegetables are rich in vitamins and minerals that help reduce inflammation.

Nuts and seeds: walnuts, almonds, flaxseeds and chia seeds are sources of omega-3 fatty acids, known for their anti-inflammatory properties.

Fatty fish: salmon, mackerel, sardines, and herring are rich in omega-3 fatty acids and are good allies in fighting inflammation.

Turmeric: This yellow-orange spice contains curcumin, a powerful anti-inflammatory compound.

Ginger: Gingerol, an active compound in ginger, has demonstrated anti-inflammatory properties.

Extra virgin olive oil: is a source of healthy fats and polyphenols, which can help reduce inflammation.

By combining these foods in our daily diet, we can promote a state of well-being and fight unwanted inflammation. In the next sections, we will explore several recipes that include these delicious anti-inflammatory ingredients. Be inspired by the variety of flavors and benefits that anti-inflammatory cooking has to offer!

Before going any further, always keep in mind that it is important to consult a health professional or nutritionist to tailor the diet to your personal needs. Each of us is unique and may need a specific diet plan. That said, let's get ready to discover how an anti-inflammatory diet can transform the way we perceive food and our overall well-being. Are you ready to dive into this healthy and tasty culinary experience?

General Guidelines for an Anti-Inflammatory Diet.

Now that we understand the key role of diet in influencing inflammation in our bodies, it is time to discover the basic guidelines for embracing an anti-inflammatory diet. Don't worry, this is not a rigid list of rules to follow to the letter, but practical advice to help you create a healthy and tasty diet that can promote your body's well-being.

1. Priority to Vegetables and Fruits.

Vegetables and fruits are the real stars of an anti-inflammatory diet. Fill your plate with a variety of dark green leafy greens, cruciferous vegetables such as cauliflower and broccoli, and antioxidant-rich seasonal fruits. These foods are rich in vitamins, minerals, and phytonutrients that help fight inflammation and keep our immune systems strong.

2. Choose Lean Protein

When it comes to protein, opt for lean, high-quality options. Fish, skinless chicken, turkey, legumes, nuts and seeds are good sources of protein that provide anti-inflammatory benefits. Limit consumption of red meat and cured meats, which can contribute to inflammation if consumed in excess.

3. Omega-3 fatty acids: A Priority.

Omega-3 fatty acids are powerful allies against inflammation. Include fatty fish such as salmon, mackerel, sardines and herring in your weekly diet. If you are vegetarian or vegan, opt for flaxseeds, chia seeds, walnuts and hemp seed oil, which are rich in omega-3s.

4. Reduce Refined Sugars and Carbohydrates.

Added sugars and refined carbohydrates can raise blood sugar levels and trigger an inflammatory response. Limit your intake of sweets, sugary drinks and foods high in white flour. Prefer whole grains such as quinoa, spelt, and oats, which contain health-beneficial nutrients.

5. Anti-inflammatory Seasonings

Incorporate anti-inflammatory seasonings such as turmeric, ginger, black pepper and extra virgin olive oil into your diet. These seasonings not only add flavor to your dishes, but also offer beneficial properties to fight inflammation.

6. Drink Water and Tea

Hydration is essential for a healthy, anti-inflammatory diet. Drink plenty of water throughout the day and enjoy green tea or herbal teas, which are rich in antioxidants, to promote proper hydration and help reduce inflammation.

7. Limit Alcohol and Coffee

Excess alcohol and caffeine can increase inflammation in our bodies. If you drink alcohol, do so in moderation, and try to balance it with increased water intake.

These guidelines are just a starting point to help you structure an anti-inflammatory diet that suits your personal needs and tastes. Be creative in the kitchen, experiment with new recipes and anti-inflammatory ingredients, and above all, listen to your body. A healthy, balanced diet is one of the keys to a healthy life without unwanted inflammation. Ready to put these guidelines into practice and discover the pleasures of anti-inflammatory eating? Then, get ready for the next sections full of delicious anti-inflammatory tips and recipes!

CHAPTER 2
The Best Natural Anti-Inflammatories: Herbs and Spices

1: Herbs and Spices that Fight Inflammation.

Herbs and spices have always played a key role in traditional cooking and natural medicine. Today, science has confirmed what the ancient traditions already knew: many herbs and spices contain powerful anti-inflammatory compounds that can help us fight inflammation in our bodies.

Here are some of the best herbs and spices that should be a valuable addition to your anti-inflammatory cooking:

1. Turmeric

Turmeric is a spice with wonderful golden hues, known for its main ingredient curcumin, a powerful anti-inflammatory compound. Curcumin can help reduce levels of pro-inflammatory cytokines in our bodies, helping to soothe inflammation. To increase the bioavailability of curcumin, combine it with a small amount of black pepper, which contains piperine, a substance that promotes curcumin absorption.

2. Ginger

Ginger is a root with a spicy and refreshing flavor that contains powerful anti-inflammatory compounds called gingerols. These compounds can help reduce inflammation and relieve pain. You can use freshly grated ginger to flavor meat, fish or vegetable dishes, or make a delicious ginger herbal tea for a soothing effect.

3. Oregano

Oregano is an aromatic herb widely used in cooking to flavor pizza, pasta, and many other dishes. It is rich in antioxidants and essential oils that have demonstrated anti-inflammatory properties. Add dried or fresh oregano to your dishes for a touch of flavor and health benefit.

4. Rosemary

Rosemary is an aromatic plant that releases an inviting fragrance. It is a source of rosmarinic acid, a compound with anti-inflammatory properties. Use rosemary to season potatoes, meats, fish or to flavor olive oil.

5. Basil

Basil is a fresh, fragrant herb that can be used in numerous recipes. It contains essential oils with anti-inflammatory properties, and pairs perfectly with fresh tomatoes, mozzarella cheese, and extra virgin olive oil for a delicious caprese salad.

6. Chili

Hot peppers are rich in capsaicin, a compound with anti-inflammatory and analgesic properties. Add some dried or fresh chili peppers to your dishes to give a jolt of flavor and help fight inflammation.

These are just some of the herbs and spices that can help reduce inflammation and improve the flavor of your preparations. Anti-inflammatory cooking can be an exciting and flavorful culinary experience in which the creative use of herbs and spices can make each dish a work of art for the palate and a panacea for the body. In the next sections, we will explore delicious recipes in which these precious herbs and spices take center stage, offering you a true sensory journey into the world of anti-inflammatory cooking!

2: Ideas and Tips for Incorporating Herbs and Spices into Recipes

Herbs and spices can transform your recipes, giving them new and enveloping flavors. In addition to their anti-inflammatory properties, these wonderful additions to your cooking will bring a touch of originality and creativity to your dishes. Let's discover together some ideas and tips for making the most of the potential of herbs and spices in preparing anti-inflammatory meals:

1. Marinades and Aromatic Sauces

Use herbs and spices to create aromatic marinades for meats, fish and vegetables. Mix extra virgin olive oil with garlic, rosemary, thyme and lemon for a succulent and anti-inflammatory chicken marinade. Make Greek yogurt-based sauces with grated ginger, turmeric and mint to accompany fish dishes or for a fresh salad.

2. Herbal teas and hot drinks

Take advantage of the beneficial properties of herbs and spices by making herbal teas and hot drinks. An infusion of ginger and turmeric with a touch of honey and lemon will give you an invigorating and anti-inflammatory drink. Also try cinnamon and star anise tea for a warm and healthy comfort drink.

3. Homemade Dry Seasonings

Make your own dry seasonings with herbs and spices, avoiding the use of prepackaged mixtures that may contain additives and preservatives. Make a mix of turmeric, black pepper, ginger and garlic powder for an anti-inflammatory powder to sprinkle on roasted vegetables or soups.

4. Fresh Herb Pestates

A basil, parsley or oregano pesto with extra virgin olive oil and walnuts is a delicious way to add flavor and nutrients to your dishes. Combine a generous amount of fresh herbs, a pinch of salt, olive oil, and walnuts or seeds to make an herb cream perfect for dressing pasta, gnocchi, or even for spreading on crostini.

5. Flavoring the Cooking Water.

When cooking grains such as rice or quinoa, add bay leaves, rosemary sprigs or cloves to the cooking water to infuse your preparations with a delicate aroma. The spices flavor the water as the grains cook, giving your dishes an enveloping flavor.

6. Fresh Gaskets

Serve your dishes with fresh herb garnishes for a touch of freshness and color. A handful of chopped parsley, basil leaves or chives can make even a simple dish like a salad or side dish a treat for the eyes and palate.

Experiment, mix and match your favorite herbs and spices to create tasty and healthy anti-inflammatory dishes. Anti-inflammatory cooking is a culinary adventure full of opportunities to express your creativity and take care of your well-being through food. In the next sections, we will delight you with recipes that highlight the harmony of anti-inflammatory herbs and spices, making your meals a tasty and beneficial experience for your health!

CHAPTER 3
The Best Anti-Inflammatory Seasonings.

1: Healthy and Anti-Inflammatory Oils and Condiments

Condiments play a vital role in cooking, adding flavor and character to our dishes. In the anti-inflammatory diet, it is important to choose seasonings that not only enhance the flavors, but also offer benefits for our health. Let's look together at some of the healthy, anti-inflammatory oils and seasonings that can become valuable allies in your cooking:

1. Extra Virgin Olive Oil

Extra virgin olive oil is a source of healthy fats, antioxidants, and monounsaturated fatty acids that can help reduce inflammation in our bodies. Use it as a base for dressing your salads, as an ingredient for marinating meats or fish, or simply for cooking vegetables in a pan. Its rich nuance of flavor and unmistakable aroma make olive oil a classic and versatile condiment.

2. Coconut Oil

Coconut oil is a condiment with a creamy texture and mild flavor. It contains medium-chain fatty acids that can support our immune system and contribute to a balanced inflammatory response. Use coconut oil to bake at high temperatures or to flavor your desserts in a healthier way.

3. Apple Vinegar

Apple cider vinegar is known for its antioxidant properties and can help stabilize blood sugar levels. Use it to dress salads or cooked vegetables for added acidity and health benefits.

4. Soy Sauce

Soy sauce is a protein- and antioxidant-rich condiment, but try to opt for the low-sodium version. Add it to your marinades, sauces or stir-fries for an umami flavor and an Asian twist to your dishes.

5. Worcestershire sauce

Worcestershire sauce is a blend of ingredients such as vinegar, molasses, and spices that offers a unique flavor to your dishes. Choose a low-sodium version and use it to season meats or flavor sauces and stews.

6. Homemade Tomato Sauce.

Make your own homemade tomato sauce using fresh tomatoes, herbs and anti-inflammatory spices such as oregano, basil and garlic. A wholesome and healthy tomato sauce to pair with whole-wheat pasta or to make delicious sauces for your dishes.

7. Basil or Arugula Pesto

A homemade pesto made with basil, arugula, walnuts, extra virgin olive oil, and cheese can be a nutritious and flavorful condiment to flavor pasta, rice, or even meat and fish.

Always remember to choose high-quality oils and seasonings, preferably organic, to maximize the health benefits and reduce the intake of unwanted additives. Use these healthy, anti-inflammatory seasonings creatively, and you will turn your dishes into true culinary works of art that satisfy the palate and nourish the body. In the next sections, we will discover recipes that make the most of the flavors of these seasonings, making your meals a delicious experience that is beneficial for overall well-being!

2: Creative Ways to Enrich Dishes with Beneficial Seasonings

Anti-inflammatory cooking offers endless possibilities for enriching dishes with beneficial seasonings, making every bite a feast for the palate and a pampering for the body. Experiment with new combinations and follow your creativity to discover the secrets of tasty and healthy cooking. Here are some creative ways to enrich your dishes with anti-inflammatory seasonings:

1. Avocado and Lime Cream

Make a delicious avocado and lime cream to accompany fish or chicken dishes. Blend ripe avocado pulp with fresh lime juice, garlic, salt and black pepper to make a smooth, refreshing cream. This sauce is rich in healthy fats, vitamins and minerals that can help fight inflammation.

2. Coconut Ginger Sauce.

Brown some grated ginger in a little coconut oil, add coconut milk and let it thicken. This creamy and aromatically spicy sauce is perfect for seasoning roasted vegetables or curry dishes.

3. Tomato Sunflower Seed Dressing.

Make a nutritious, anti-inflammatory dressing by blending toasted sunflower seeds, sun-dried tomatoes, fresh basil, garlic, extra virgin olive oil, and a splash of apple cider vinegar. This dressing can be used to flavor pasta, salads or as a spread for croutons.

4. Quinoa Salad with Soy Sauce and Ginger.

Prepare a quinoa salad with crunchy vegetables and dress with a vinaigrette made from soy sauce, grated ginger, sesame oil and garlic. This combination of Asian flavors is both tasty and anti-inflammatory.

5. Chickpea Chili Hummus

Make your own chickpea hummus at home, adding dried red pepper for a spicy, anti-inflammatory kick. This healthy and nutritious hummus can be used as a topping for sandwiches, crackers, or as a dip for raw vegetables.

6. Guacamole with Turmeric and Black Pepper.

Enrich traditional guacamole with a sprinkling of turmeric and black pepper. This combination will give guacamole not only an enveloping flavor but also anti-inflammatory properties.

7. Cinnamon Sauce for Sweets.

Prepare a sweet sauce made with cinnamon, honey and Greek yogurt to accompany healthy, anti-inflammatory desserts such as fresh fruit or fruit-based desserts.

Take advantage of these creative and beneficial seasonings to turn every meal into a memorable and healthy dining experience. Anti-inflammatory cooking allows you to discover new flavor combinations and take care of your body through food. In the next sections, we will guide you in preparing extraordinary dishes that will best employ the powers of these beneficial seasonings for a table full of taste and health!

CHAPTER 4
The Best Anti-Inflammatory Foods Present at the Supermarket and Which Ones to Absolutely Avoid

1: The Anti-Inflammatory Shopping List.

Your shopping list is a powerful tool for creating a balanced and tasty anti-inflammatory diet. When you visit the supermarket, focus on foods rich in anti-inflammatory properties and limit those that can contribute to inflammation in the body. Here is a guide to help you make smart choices in your grocery shopping:

1. Fresh Fruit

Opt for fruits that are fresh, colorful and rich in antioxidants. Apples, berries, citrus fruits, cherries and pomegranates are just some of the examples of anti-inflammatory fruits to include on your shopping list.

2. Green Leafy Vegetables.

Green leafy vegetables, such as spinach, kale and arugula, are rich in vitamins, minerals and antioxidant compounds that can help fight inflammation. Include these vegetables in your cart for a nutritious and tasty anti-inflammatory diet.

3. Dried Fruits and Nuts.

Walnuts, almonds, hazelnuts, and Brazil nuts are rich in healthy fats and antioxidants, which can help reduce inflammation. Use them as a snack or as an ingredient to enrich salads and main dishes.

4. Fatty Fish

Salmon, sardines, herring and mackerel are examples of fatty fish rich in omega-3 fatty acids, known for their anti-inflammatory properties. Include fatty fish in your diet at least twice a week to take advantage of their benefits.

5. Legumes

Legumes, such as chickpeas, beans, lentils and peas, are sources of plant protein and fiber, which can help stabilize blood sugar levels and reduce inflammation. Add legumes to your dishes for a touch of flavor and nutrition.

6. Whole grain cereals

Prefer whole grains, such as brown rice, quinoa, spelt and oats, which are rich in fiber and nutrients that can contribute to an anti-inflammatory diet.

7. Healthy Oils

Choose extra virgin olive oil, coconut oil, and flaxseed oil for cooking and cold preparations. These oils contain healthy fats and antioxidant compounds that promote a balanced inflammatory response in the body.

8. Anti-inflammatory Spices

Add spices such as turmeric, ginger, cinnamon, oregano and black pepper to your shopping list. These spices are rich in compounds with anti-inflammatory properties and can be easily incorporated into many recipes.

Use this shopping list as a guide to create healthy, anti-inflammatory meals by choosing foods that nourish your body and support your overall well-being. With a balanced and conscious shopping list, you can bring tasty, anti-inflammatory cuisine to the table that will make you feel your best!

2: Foods to Avoid to Reduce Inflammation in the Body.

In your quest for an anti-inflammatory diet, it is equally important to identify and reduce the consumption of foods that may contribute to inflammation in the body. Avoiding some unhealthy food choices can be key to promoting better management of inflammation. Here are some foods that are best limited or avoided:

1. Refined Sugars and Artificial Sweeteners.

Refined sugars, such as those found in sugary drinks, packaged sweets and high-sugar foods, can trigger blood sugar spikes, increasing the risk of inflammation and metabolic imbalances. Also avoid excessive use of artificial sweeteners, which can have long-term adverse health effects.

2. Saturated Fats and Trans Fats.

Saturated fats, found mainly in fatty meats, whole dairy products and some vegetable oils such as coconut oil, can contribute to inflammation if consumed in excess. Trans fats, commonly found in fried foods, industrial baked goods, and packaged foods, are also known to have adverse health effects and can increase the level of inflammation in the body.

3. Processed Meat

Processed meats, such as cured meats, sausages, bacon, and pre-cooked hamburgers, often contain high amounts of sodium, preservatives, and unhealthy fats. These foods can trigger inflammatory responses in our bodies and are best avoided or consumed in moderation.

4. Fried Foods and Salty Snacks

Fried foods, such as French fries, fried chicken and onion rings, are often high in saturated and trans fats, which can contribute to inflammation. In addition, salty snacks such as chips and crackers often contain high amounts of sodium and unhealthy fats, so it is best to limit their consumption.

5. Alcohol

Excessive alcohol consumption can increase inflammation in the body and have negative effects on overall health. Limit alcohol consumption and try to prefer drinks in moderation.

6. High Sodium Foods.

Some foods such as convenience foods, salty snacks, packaged sauces and canned foods can be high in sodium. Excessive sodium in the diet can promote water retention and inflammation. Read food labels carefully and try to choose low-sodium foods.

7. Highly Processed Foods

Avoid highly processed foods, such as packaged foods, ready-to-eat meals, fast-foods, and industrial baked goods. These foods may contain additives, preservatives and unhealthy ingredients that can increase inflammation and have negative effects on long-term health.

By reducing or avoiding these unhealthy foods and focusing on a diet rich in anti-inflammatory foods, you can help support your overall well-being and promote better management of inflammation in the body. Being aware of your food choices can make a difference in your long-term health and well-being.

CHAPTER 5
Recipes

1: Anti-Inflammatory Breakfasts

1. Kiwi and Spinach Smoothie

Ingredients for 2 persons:

:

- o 2 ripe kiwis, peeled and cut into pieces
- o 1 cup of fresh spinach
- o 1 ripe banana
- o 1 cup of unsweetened almond milk
- o 1 teaspoon turmeric powder
- o 1 teaspoon fresh grated ginger
- o 1 teaspoon honey (optional for sweetening)

Instructions:

1. Place all ingredients in the blender except the honey, if used.
2. Blend until smooth and creamy.
3. Taste and, if necessary, sweeten with honey.
4. Serve in a glass and garnish with a few spinach leaves or a slice of kiwi.

2. Avocado Toast with Fried Egg.

Ingredients for 2 persons:

- o 1 ripe avocado, peeled and mashed
- o 2 slices of toasted whole wheat bread
- o 2 fresh eggs
- o Freshly ground black pepper
- o Sea salt
- o 1 teaspoon of extra virgin olive oil
- o Smoked paprika (optional)

Instructions:

1. Heat extra virgin olive oil in a nonstick skillet over medium heat.
2. Add the eggs to the pan and cook them sunny side up, adding salt and black pepper to taste.
3. Spread the mashed avocado on the toasted bread slices.
4. Arrange the fried eggs on the slices of bread with the avocado.
5. Sprinkle with smoked paprika (if desired) for extra flavor.

3. Oatmeal Porridge with Berries.

1 Ingredients for 2 persons:

- o 1 cup of oatmeal
- o 2 cups of unsweetened almond milk
- o 1 cup of mixed berries (strawberries, blueberries, raspberries)
- o 1 teaspoon cinnamon powder
- o 1 teaspoon honey (optional for sweetening)

Instructions:

1. In a saucepan, bring the almond milk to a boil.
2. Add the oatmeal and mix well.
3. Reduce the heat and cook over medium-low heat for 5-7 minutes, stirring occasionally.
4. Turn off the heat and let it rest for a minute.

5. Transfer the porridge to two bowls and add the berries on top.
6. Sprinkle with cinnamon and, if desired, sweeten with honey.

4. Banana and Walnut Pancakes

Ingredients for 2 persons:

- o   1 ripe banana, mashed
- o   2 eggs
- o   1/2 cup oatmeal
- o   1 teaspoon baking powder
- o   1/4 cup chopped walnuts
- o   1/2 teaspoon cinnamon powder
- o   Coconut oil to grease the pan

Instructions:

1. In a bowl, mix together the mashed banana and eggs.
2. Add the oat flour, baking powder, and cinnamon and mix until smooth.
3. Add chopped walnuts and mix.
4. Heat some coconut oil in a nonstick skillet over medium heat.
5. Pour some of the batter into the pan and cook the pancakes until golden brown on both sides.
6. Serve the pancakes hot with a sprinkle of cinnamon and a sliced banana.

5. Almond Butter and Raspberry Jam on Whole Wheat Bread.

Ingredients for 2 persons:

- o   2 slices of whole wheat bread
- o   Natural almond butter (no added sugar)
- o   Raspberry jam with no added sugar

Instructions:

1. Toast the slices of whole-wheat bread.
2. Spread one slice of bread with almond butter and the other with raspberry jam.

3. Combine the two slices to form a delicious anti-inflammatory sandwich.

6. Omelette with Herbs and Cherry Tomatoes.

Ingredients for 2 persons:

- o   4 eggs
- o   1/4 cup of unsweetened almond milk
- o   1/2 cup cherry tomatoes cut in half
- o   1 red onion, sliced
- o   1 handful of fresh basil leaves
- o   1 tablespoon of olive oil
- o   Sea salt and black pepper to taste

Instructions:

1. In a bowl, beat the eggs with the almond milk, salt and pepper.
2. Heat olive oil in a nonstick skillet over medium heat.
3. Add onion and cook until soft.
4. Add the cherry tomatoes and cook for a few minutes until they become soft.
5. Pour the beaten eggs into the pan with the vegetables.
6. Add fresh basil leaves.
7. Cook the omelet until it is well set.
8. Cut into wedges and serve hot.

7. Egg Burrito with Avocado and Tomato Sauce.

Ingredients for 2 persons:

- o   2 eggs
- o   1 ripe avocado, cut into slices
- o   2 corn or whole wheat tortillas
- o   1/2 cup homemade tomato sauce (no added sugar)

1. Beat the eggs in a bowl and cook them in a nonstick skillet over medium-low heat until well cooked.
2. Heat the tortillas slightly in a frying pan or in the microwave.
3. Spread the eggs on the tortillas and add the avocado slices.
4. Roll the tortillas to form burritos.
5. Serve with tomato sauce to use as a dressing.

8. Yogurt, Fruit and Homemade Granola Parfait.

Ingredients for 2 persons:

- 1 cup of natural Greek yogurt (no added sugar)
- 1/2 cup mixed berries (strawberries, blueberries, raspberries)
- 1/4 cup homemade granola (no added sugars)

Instructions:

1. In a glass or bowl, alternate layers of Greek yogurt, berries and homemade granola.
2. Continue forming layers until you run out of ingredients.
3. Finish with a layer of granola on top.
4. Serve as a delicious anti-inflammatory parfait.

9. Apple Cinnamon Muffins.

Ingredients for 2 persons:

- 1 1/2 cups of oatmeal
- 1 teaspoon baking powder
- 1/2 teaspoon baking soda
- 1/4 teaspoon of sea salt
- 1 teaspoon cinnamon powder
- 1/2 cup unsweetened almond milk
- 1/4 cup of melted coconut oil
- 1/4 cup of honey
- 1 egg
- 1 large apple, peeled and grated

Instructions:

1. Preheat the oven to 350°F and line a muffin pan with paper cups.
2. In a bowl, mix the oat flour, baking powder, baking soda, cinnamon, and salt.
3. In another bowl, mix the almond milk, melted coconut oil, honey and egg.
4. Combine the wet ingredients with the dry ingredients and mix until smooth.
5. Add the grated apple and mix well.
6. Spread the batter into the paper ramekins.
7. Bake the muffins in the oven for about 15 to 18 minutes or until they are golden brown on the surface.
8. Bake and allow to cool slightly before serving.

10. Sweet Potato Toast with Avocado Cream.

Ingredients for 2 persons:

- 2 medium sweet potatoes, thinly sliced
- 1 ripe avocado, crushed
- Juice of half a lemon
- Sea salt and black pepper to taste
- Chia seeds (optional for garnish)

Instructions:

1. Heat a grill or nonstick skillet over medium heat.
2. Grill the sweet potato slices until tender and lightly browned on both sides.
3. In a bowl, mash the avocado and add the lemon juice, salt and pepper.
4. Blend until smooth.

5. Spread the avocado cream on the grilled sweet potato slices.
6. Garnish with chia seeds (if desired) for a touch of crunch.

11. Whole Wheat Waffles with Fresh Fruit and Maple Syrup.

Ingredients for 2 persons:

- o 1 cup of whole wheat flour
- o 1 tablespoon of coconut sugar
- o 2 teaspoons baking powder
- o 1/4 teaspoon of sea salt
- o 1 cup of unsweetened almond milk
- o 2 tablespoons of melted coconut oil
- o 1 egg
- o Fresh fruit of your choice (strawberries, blueberries, bananas)
- o Pure maple syrup (no added sugar)

Instructions:

1. Preheat the waffle maker according to the manufacturer's instructions.
2. In a bowl, mix the whole wheat flour, coconut sugar, baking powder, and salt.
3. In another bowl, mix the almond milk, melted coconut oil and egg.
4. Combine the wet ingredients with the dry ingredients and mix until smooth.
5. Pour the batter into the waffle maker and bake until the waffles are golden brown and crispy.
6. Serve waffles with fresh fruit and maple syrup to taste.

12. Smoothie Bowl with Acai and Coconut

Ingredients for 2 persons:

- o 1 package of frozen acai pulp
- o 1 ripe banana
- o 1/2 cup unsweetened coconut milk
- o 1 tablespoon almond butter
- o Fresh fruit of your choice (blueberries, raspberries, kiwi)
- o Grated coconut (no added sugars)
- o Homemade granola (no added sugars)

Instructions:

1. In a blender, blend the acai pulp, banana, coconut milk, and almond butter until smooth.
2. Pour the smoothie into a bowl.
3. Garnish with fresh fruit, grated coconut and homemade granola.

13. Scrambled Eggs with Asparagus and Cherry Tomatoes.

Ingredients for 2 persons:

- o 4 eggs
- o 1/4 cup of unsweetened almond milk
- o 1 bunch of fresh asparagus, cut into pieces
- o 1 cup cherry tomatoes, cut in half
- o 1 red onion, sliced
- o 1 tablespoon of olive oil
- o Sea salt and black pepper to taste

Instructions:

1. Heat olive oil in a nonstick skillet over medium heat.
2. Add onion and cook until soft.
3. Add asparagus and cherry tomatoes and cook for a few minutes until tender.
4. In a bowl, beat the eggs with the almond milk, salt and pepper.
5. Pour the eggs into the pan with the vegetables.
6. Cook, stirring gently, until eggs are well scrambled and cooked to your liking.
7. Serve hot.

14. Whole Wheat Banana Bread with Walnuts

Ingredients for 2 persons:

- o 1 1/2 cups whole-wheat flour
- o 1 teaspoon baking powder
- o 1/2 teaspoon baking soda
- o 1/4 teaspoon of sea salt
- o 3 ripe bananas, mashed
- o 1/4 cup of melted coconut oil
- o 1/4 cup of honey
- o 1/4 cup of unsweetened almond milk
- o 1 egg
- o 1/2 cup chopped walnuts

Instructions:

1. Preheat the oven to 350°F and line a loaf pan with baking paper.
2. In a bowl, mix the whole wheat flour, baking powder, baking soda, and salt.
3. In another bowl, mix the mashed bananas, melted coconut oil, honey, almond milk, and egg.
4. Combine the wet ingredients with the dry ingredients and mix until smooth.
5. Add chopped walnuts and mix well.
6. Pour the dough into the baking dish and level the surface.
7. Bake for about 45-50 minutes or until a toothpick inserted in the center comes out clean.
8. Let the banana bread cool before cutting it into slices.

15. Buckwheat Crepes with Berries.

Ingredients for 2 persons:

- o 1 cup buckwheat flour
- o 1/4 teaspoon of sea salt
- o 2 eggs
- o 1 1/4 cups of unsweetened almond milk
- o 1 teaspoon of melted coconut oil
- o Mixed berries (strawberries, blueberries, raspberries)
- o Pure maple syrup (no added sugar)

Instructions:

1. In a bowl, mix buckwheat flour and salt.
2. In another bowl, beat the eggs with the almond milk and melted coconut oil.
3. Combine the wet ingredients with the dry ingredients and mix until a smooth batter is obtained.
4. Heat a nonstick skillet over medium heat and lightly grease it with melted coconut oil.
5. Pour a ladleful of batter into the pan and cook the crepe until it is golden brown on both sides.
6. Repeat the process with the rest of the batter.
7. Serve the crepes with the berries and maple syrup.

16. Anti-inflammatory Green Smoothie

Ingredients for 2 persons:

- o 1 cup of fresh spinach
- o 1 cup fresh kale
- o 1/2 ripe avocado
- o 1/2 ripe banana
- o 1/2 cup unsweetened coconut water
- o Juice of half a lemon
- o 1 teaspoon fresh grated ginger
- o Ice to taste

Instructions:

1. In a blender, blend the spinach, kale, avocado, banana, coconut water, lemon juice, and ginger until smooth.
2. Add ice and blend until smoothie is well chilled and smooth.
3. Pour into a glass and serve immediately.

17. Zucchini and Peppers Omelette.

Ingredients for 2 persons:

- 4 eggs
- 1/4 cup of unsweetened almond milk
- 1 large zucchini, cut into thin rounds
- 1 red bell pepper, cut into strips
- 1 red onion, sliced
- 1 tablespoon of olive oil
- Sea salt and black pepper to taste

Instructions:

1. In a bowl, beat the eggs with the almond milk, salt and pepper.
2. Heat olive oil in a nonstick skillet over medium heat.
3. Add onion and cook until soft.
4. Add the zucchini and peppers and cook for a few minutes until tender.
5. Pour the beaten eggs into the pan with the vegetables.
6. Cook, stirring gently, until the eggs are well set.
7. Cut into wedges and serve hot.

18. Quinoa Porridge with Dried Fruit.

Ingredients for 2 persons:

- 1 cup of quinoa
- 2 cups of unsweetened almond milk
- 1/4 teaspoon cinnamon powder
- 1/4 cup sliced almonds
- 1/4 cup chopped pecans
- Mixed dried fruits (raisins, dried apricots, dates)

Instructions:

1. Rinse the quinoa under running water.
2. In a saucepan, bring the almond milk to a boil.
3. Add the quinoa and cinnamon and reduce the heat to medium-low.
4. Cover and cook for about 15 to 20 minutes or until the quinoa is cooked and the liquid has been absorbed.
5. Lightly toast sliced almonds and pecans in a dry frying pan.
6. Serve the quinoa porridge with the toasted nuts on top.

19. Pumpkin Pancakes with Chia Seeds.

Ingredients for 2 persons:

- 1 cup whole wheat flour
- 1 teaspoon baking powder
- 1/2 teaspoon baking soda
- 1/4 teaspoon of sea salt
- 1 cup of pumpkin puree
- 1 cup of unsweetened almond milk
- 2 tablespoons of melted coconut oil
- 1 tablespoon of chia seeds

Instructions:

1. In a bowl, mix the whole wheat flour, baking powder, baking soda, and salt.
2. In another bowl, mix the pumpkin puree, almond milk, and melted coconut oil.
3. Combine the wet ingredients with the dry ingredients and mix until a smooth batter is obtained.
4. Heat a nonstick skillet over medium heat and lightly grease it with melted coconut oil.
5. Pour a ladleful of batter into the pan and cook the pancake until golden brown on both sides.
6. Continue cooking the rest of the batter.
7. Sprinkle the pancakes with chia seeds before serving.

20. Coconut and Pineapple Smoothie

Ingredients for 2 persons:

- 1 cup unsweetened coconut milk
- 1 cup diced fresh pineapple

- 1/2 ripe banana
- 1 tablespoon grated coconut (no added sugar)
- Ice to taste

Instructions:

1. In a blender, blend the coconut milk, pineapple, banana, and grated coconut until smooth.
2. Add ice and blend until smoothie is well chilled and smooth.
3. Pour into a glass and serve immediately.

2: Healthy and nutritious cues

21. Chickpea Hummus with Vegetable Crudités.

Ingredients for 2 persons:

- 1 can of rinsed and drained chickpeas
- Juice of 1 lemon
- 2 tablespoons of tahini (sesame seed cream)
- 2 tablespoons of extra virgin olive oil
- 1 clove of garlic
- 1/4 teaspoon cumin powder
- Sea salt and black pepper to taste
- Carrots, celery and peppers for crudités

Instructions:

1. In a blender, blend the chickpeas, lemon juice, tahini, olive oil, garlic, cumin, salt, and pepper until smooth.
2. Serve the hummus with the vegetable crudités.

22. Quinoa and avocado salad.

Ingredients for 2 persons:

- 1 cup of cooked quinoa
- 1 ripe avocado, cut into cubes
- 1/2 cucumber, diced
- 1/4 red onion, thinly sliced
- 1 tablespoon sunflower seeds
- Juice of 1 lime
- 1 tablespoon of extra virgin olive oil
- Sea salt and black pepper to taste

Instructions:

1. In a bowl, mix the cooked quinoa, avocado, cucumber, and red onion.
2. Season with lime juice, olive oil, salt and pepper.
3. Sprinkle with sunflower seeds before serving.

23. Guacamole with Corn Tortilla.

Ingredients for 2 persons:

- 2 ripe avocados, crushed
- 1 ripe tomato, diced
- 1/4 red onion, thinly sliced
- Juice of 1 lime
- Chopped fresh coriander
- Sea salt and black pepper to taste
- Corn tortilla to accompany

Instructions:

1. In a bowl, mix the mashed avocados, tomato, red onion, lime juice, and cilantro.
2. Season with salt and pepper to taste.
3. Serve the guacamole with the corn tortillas.

24. Grilled Eggplant with Lentil Hummus.

Ingredients for 2 persons:

- 2 eggplants, thinly sliced
- Extra virgin olive oil
- Sea salt and black pepper to taste
- 1 can of rinsed and drained lentils
- 2 tablespoons of extra virgin olive oil
- Juice of 1 lemon
- 1 clove of garlic
- Smoked paprika
- Chopped fresh parsley

Instructions:

1. Brush the eggplant slices with olive oil and season with salt and pepper.
2. Grill the eggplant until soft and well scored from the grill.
3. In a blender, blend the lentils, olive oil, lemon juice, garlic, salt, pepper, and paprika until smooth.
4. Serve the grilled eggplant with the lentil hummus and sprinkle with fresh parsley.

25. Wholewheat Carrot Walnut Muffins.

Ingredients for 2 persons:

- 1 cup of whole wheat flour
- 1/2 cup coconut sugar
- 1 teaspoon baking powder
- 1/2 teaspoon baking soda
- 1/4 teaspoon of sea salt
- 1 teaspoon cinnamon powder
- 1/4 cup of melted coconut oil
- 1/4 cup of unsweetened almond milk
- 2 eggs
- 1 cup grated carrots
- 1/2 cup chopped walnuts

Instructions:

1. Preheat the oven to 350°F (about 180°C) and prepare a muffin pan with paper cups.
2. In a bowl, mix the whole wheat flour, coconut sugar, baking powder, baking soda, salt, and cinnamon.
3. In another bowl, mix the melted coconut oil, almond milk and eggs.
4. Combine the wet ingredients with the dry ingredients and mix until smooth.
5. Add grated carrots and chopped walnuts and mix well.
6. Pour the batter into the paper ramekins, filling them about 2/3 full.
7. Bake for about 15 to 18 minutes or until a toothpick inserted in the center comes out clean.
8. Let the muffins cool before enjoying them.

26. Guacamole Sauce with Baked Corn Chips.

Ingredients for 2 persons:

- 2 ripe avocados, crushed
- 1 ripe tomato, diced
- 1/4 red onion, thinly sliced
- Juice of 1 lime
- Chopped fresh coriander
- Sea salt and black pepper to taste
- Baked whole corn chips to accompany

Instructions:

1. In a bowl, mix the mashed avocados, tomato, red onion, lime juice, and cilantro.
2. Season with salt and pepper to taste.
3. Serve the guacamole sauce with baked whole corn chips.

27. Coconut Mango Smoothie

Ingredients for 2 persons:

- 1 cup of unsweetened coconut milk
- 1 cup diced fresh mango
- 1/2 ripe banana
- 1 tablespoon grated coconut (no added sugar)
- Ice to taste

Instructions:

1. In a blender, blend the coconut milk, mango, banana, and grated coconut until smooth.
2. Add ice and blend until smoothie is well chilled and smooth.
3. Pour into a glass and serve immediately.

28. Sweet Potato Crostini with Guacamole.

Ingredients for 2 persons:

- 2 medium sweet potatoes, thinly sliced
- Extra virgin olive oil
- Sea salt and black pepper to taste
- 2 ripe avocados, crushed
- 1 ripe tomato, diced
- 1/4 red onion, thinly sliced
- Juice of 1 lime
- Chopped fresh coriander

Instructions:

1. Preheat the oven to 375°F (about 190°C) and line a baking sheet with baking paper.
2. Brush the sweet potato slices with olive oil and season with salt and pepper.
3. Arrange the sweet potato slices on the baking sheet and bake them in the oven until soft and slightly crispy.
4. In a bowl, mix crushed avocados, tomato, red onion, lime juice, and cilantro to make guacamole.

5. Spread the guacamole on the sweet potato slices and serve as croutons.

29. Blueberry and Banana Smoothie

Ingredients for 2 persons:

- 1 cup of unsweetened almond milk
- 1 cup of fresh or frozen blueberries
- 1 ripe banana
- 1 tablespoon of flaxseed
- Ice to taste

Instructions:

1. In a blender, blend the almond milk, blueberries, banana, and flaxseed until smooth.
2. Add ice and blend until smoothie is well chilled and smooth.
3. Pour into a glass and serve immediately.

30. Chickpea and Tomato Salad

Ingredients for 2 persons:

- 1 can of rinsed and drained chickpeas
- 1 cup of cherry tomatoes cut in half
- 1/4 red onion, thinly sliced
- 2 tablespoons of extra virgin olive oil
- Juice of 1 lemon
- Chopped fresh parsley
- Sea salt and black pepper to taste

Instructions:

1. In a bowl, mix the chickpeas, cherry tomatoes, red onion, olive oil, and lemon juice.
2. Season with fresh chopped parsley, salt and pepper to taste.
3. Allow to season in the refrigerator for at least 30 minutes before serving.

31. Chicken and Avocado Wrap

Ingredients for 2 persons:

- o   1 whole-wheat tortilla
- o   ounces of chicken breast cooked and thinly sliced
- o   1/2 ripe avocado, sliced
- o   Mixed salad
- o   Yogurt and lemon sauce (Greek yogurt, lemon juice, garlic, salt and pepper)

Instructions:

1. Heat the whole-wheat tortilla in a lightly greased skillet.
2. Spread the chicken breast slices on the tortilla.
3. Add the avocado slices and mixed salad.
4. Roll up the tortilla to form a wrap and cut it in half.
5. Serve with the yogurt and lemon sauce.

32. Curry and Turmeric Popcorn.

Ingredients for 2 persons:

- o   1/2 cup unsalted popcorn
- o   1 teaspoon of melted coconut oil
- o   1 teaspoon curry powder
- o   1/2 teaspoon turmeric powder
- o   Sea salt to taste

Instructions:

1. Popcorn in microwave oven according to instructions on package.
2. In a bowl, mix the melted coconut oil, curry, turmeric, and salt.
3. Pour the seasoning mix over the hot popcorn and mix well.

33. Baked Crispy Chickpeas

Ingredients for 2 persons:

- o   1 can of rinsed and drained chickpeas
- o   1 tablespoon extra virgin olive oil
- o   1 teaspoon paprika
- o   1/2 teaspoon garlic powder
- o   1/2 teaspoon black pepper
- o   1/2 teaspoon of sea salt

Instructions:

1. Preheat the oven to 400°F (about 200°C) and line a baking sheet with baking paper.
2. In a bowl, mix the chickpeas, olive oil, paprika, garlic powder, black pepper, and salt until the chickpeas are well seasoned.
3. Arrange the chickpeas on the baking sheet in a single layer.
4. Bake in the oven for about 25-30 minutes or until the chickpeas are crispy.
5. Let them cool before enjoying.

34. Carrots with Beet Hummus.

Ingredients for 2 persons:

- o   2 medium carrots, cut into sticks
- o   1/2 cooked and diced beet
- o   1 can of rinsed and drained chickpeas
- o   2 tablespoons of tahini (sesame seed cream)
- o   Juice of 1 lemon
- o   1 clove of garlic
- o   2 tablespoons of extra virgin olive oil
- o   Sea salt and black pepper to taste

Instructions:

1. In a blender, blend the beet, chickpeas, tahini, lemon juice, garlic clove, olive oil, salt and pepper until smooth.
2. Pour the beet hummus into a bowl.
3. Accompany the carrots with beet hummus.

35. Walnut and Dried Fruit Mix.

Ingredients for 2 persons:

- o 1/4 cup pecans
- o 1/4 cup of Brazil nuts
- o 1/4 cup of almonds
- o 1/4 cup of walnuts
- o 1/4 cup of raisins

Instructions:

1. Mix all the nuts and dried fruits in a bowl.
2. Serve as a mix of dried fruits and nuts for an energy snack.

36. Smoked Salmon and Avocado Cream Roll-Up.

Ingredients for 2 persons:

- o 2 slices of smoked salmon
- o 1/2 ripe avocado, mashed
- o Juice of 1 lemon
- o Ground black pepper and sea salt to taste
- o Mixed salad

Instructions:

1. In a bowl, mix mashed avocado with lemon juice, black pepper, and salt.
2. Spread the crushed avocado over the slices of smoked salmon.
3. Add some mixed salad.
4. Roll up the salmon to form a roll-up and enjoy it as a healthy snack.

37. Orange and Ginger Smoothie.

Ingredients for 2 persons:

- o 1 cup of freshly squeezed orange juice
- o 1 ripe banana
- o 1/2-inch fresh ginger, peeled and grated
- o 1 tablespoon raw honey (optional)

- o Ice to taste

Instructions:

1. In a blender, blend the orange juice, banana, ginger and honey (if desired) until smooth.
2. Add ice and blend until smoothie is well chilled and smooth.
3. Pour into a glass and serve immediately.

38. Fresh Fruit Skewers

Ingredients for 2 persons:

- o 1 banana, cut into thick slices
- o 1/2 pineapple, diced
- o 1 apple, diced
- o 1/2 cup strawberries, cut in half
- o 1/2 cup of seedless grapes

Instructions:

1. Thread the fruit pieces onto skewers.
2. Serve the skewers with fresh fruit for a light and sweet snack.

39. Wholemeal Bread Croutons with Avocado and Dried Tomatoes.

Ingredients for 2 persons:

- o 4 slices of whole wheat bread
- o 1 ripe avocado, crushed
- o 4 sun-dried tomatoes in oil, chopped
- o Ground black pepper and sea salt to taste
- o Chopped fresh basil

Instructions:

1. Toast the slices of whole-wheat bread.
2. Spread the mashed avocado on the toasted bread slices.
3. Add the chopped sun-dried tomatoes.
4. Season with black pepper, sea salt and fresh basil.

5. Cut the croutons in half and serve as a tasty snack.

40. Baked Zucchini Fries

Ingredients for 2 persons:

- 2 medium zucchini, thinly sliced
- 2 tablespoons of extra virgin olive oil
- 1/2 teaspoon paprika
- 1/2 teaspoon garlic powder
- Sea salt and black pepper to taste

Instructions:

1. Preheat the oven to 375°F (about 190°C) and line a baking sheet with baking paper.
2. In a bowl, mix zucchini slices with olive oil, paprika, garlic powder, salt and pepper.
3. Arrange the zucchini slices on the baking sheet in a single layer.
4. Bake for about 15-20 minutes or until zucchini chips are crispy.
5. Let them cool before enjoying.

3: Balanced and Delicious Lunches.

41. Quinoa Salad with Grilled Vegetables.

Ingredients for 2 persons:

- 1 cup of cooked quinoa
- 1 zucchini, thinly sliced
- 1 red bell pepper, cut into strips
- 1 carrot, thinly sliced
- 1 red onion, thinly sliced
- 2 tablespoons of extra virgin olive oil
- Juice of 1 lemon
- 1 clove of garlic, minced
- Sea salt and black pepper to taste
- Mixed salad

Instructions:

1. Heat a grill and cook zucchini slices, bell bell pepper strips, carrot slices, and sliced onions until tender and slightly charred.
2. In a bowl, mix the cooked quinoa with the grilled vegetables.
3. Prepare a vinaigrette with the olive oil, lemon juice, garlic clove, salt and pepper.
4. Dress the salad with the vinaigrette and serve with mixed salad.

42. Chicken Curry with Vegetables and Brown Rice.

Ingredients for 2 persons:

- 2 chicken breasts, cut into cubes
- 1 onion, thinly sliced
- 1 yellow bell pepper, cut into strips
- 1 zucchini, thinly sliced
- 2 tablespoons of red curry paste
- 1 can of coconut milk
- 1 cup fresh or frozen peas
- 2 cups of cooked brown rice

Instructions:

1. In a nonstick skillet, cook the chicken cubes until golden brown.
2. Add the onion, bell bell pepper, and zucchini and cook until tender.
3. Add the curry paste and mix well.
4. Pour in the coconut milk and add the peas.
5. Continue cooking until the chicken and vegetables are fully cooked and the sauce is thick and creamy.
6. Serve the chicken curry with the cooked brown rice.

43. Grilled Salmon with Asparagus and Sweet Potatoes.

Ingredients for 2 persons:

- 2 salmon fillets
- 1 bunch of asparagus
- 2 medium sweet potatoes, diced
- 2 tablespoons of extra virgin olive oil
- Juice of 1 lemon
- 1 tablespoon chopped fresh thyme
- Sea salt and black pepper to taste

Instructions:

1. Heat a grill and cook the salmon fillets until well roasted.
2. In a bowl, mix the asparagus and sweet potatoes with the olive oil, lemon juice, and thyme.
3. Cook vegetables on the grill until tender and slightly charred.
4. Season the salmon and vegetables with salt and pepper to taste and serve.

44. Lentil and Vegetable Soup.

Ingredients for 2 persons:

- 1 cup dried red lentils
- 1 onion, thinly sliced
- 2 carrots, diced
- 2 celery stalks, thinly sliced
- 2 cloves of garlic, minced
- 1 can of diced tomatoes
- 4 cups of vegetable broth
- 1 tablespoon extra virgin olive oil
- 1 teaspoon cumin powder
- 1/2 teaspoon turmeric powder
- Sea salt and black pepper to taste
- Chopped fresh parsley

Instructions:

1. Heat olive oil in a pot and cook the onion, carrots, celery, and garlic until tender.

2. Add the dried lentils, diced tomatoes, vegetable broth, cumin, and turmeric.
3. Bring to a boil and reduce to medium-low heat. Simmer until the lentils are soft and the soup is thick and creamy.
4. Season with salt and pepper to taste and serve with fresh chopped parsley.

45. Vegetarian Wrap with Hummus

Ingredients for 2 persons:

- 2 whole-wheat tortillas
- 1 cup hummus (or use the chickpea hummus recipe from the previous subchapters)
- 1 cup of mixed salad
- 1/2 cucumber, thinly sliced
- 1/2 ripe avocado, sliced
- 1/2 red bell pepper, cut into strips

Instructions:

1. Heat whole-wheat tortillas in a lightly greased skillet.
2. Spread the hummus on the tortillas.
3. Add the mixed salad, cucumber slices, sliced avocado, and bell bell pepper strips.
4. Roll the tortillas to form wraps and cut them in half.
5. Serve vegetarian wraps with hummus as a healthy and light lunch.

46. Quinoa Salad with Avocado and Black Beans.

Ingredients for 2 persons:

- 1 cup of cooked quinoa
- 1 ripe avocado, sliced
- 1 can of black beans, rinsed and drained
- 1/2 cup sweet corn (fresh or frozen)
- 1/4 cup red onion, thinly sliced
- Juice of 1 lime
- 2 tablespoons of extra virgin olive oil

- Chopped fresh coriander
- Sea salt and black pepper to taste

Instructions:

1. In a bowl, mix cooked quinoa with sliced avocado, black beans, corn, and red onion.
2. Prepare a vinaigrette with the lime juice, olive oil, salt and pepper.
3. Dress the salad with the vinaigrette and sprinkle with chopped fresh cilantro.

47. Lemon and Rosemary Chicken with Roasted Potatoes.

Ingredients for 2 persons:

- 2 chicken breasts
- 2 lemons, one squeezed and the other sliced
- 2 tablespoons of extra virgin olive oil
- 2 cloves of garlic, minced
- 1 sprig of fresh rosemary
- 4 potatoes, diced
- Sea salt and black pepper to taste

Instructions:

1. In a bowl, mix the lemon juice, olive oil, minced garlic, and rosemary leaves.
2. Marinate the chicken breasts in the lemon-rosemary mixture for at least 30 minutes.
3. Heat a skillet and cook the chicken breasts until golden brown and cooked through.
4. Meanwhile, preheat the oven to 400°F (about 200°C) and line a baking sheet with baking paper.
5. In a bowl, mix potato cubes with olive oil, salt, and pepper.
6. Arrange the potatoes on the baking sheet in a single layer and bake them until golden brown and crispy.

7. Serve the lemon chicken with the roasted potatoes.

48. Quinoa and Bean Burrito with Guacamole.

Ingredients for 2 persons:

- 1 cup of cooked quinoa
- 1 can of black beans, rinsed and drained
- 1/2 cup sweet corn (fresh or frozen)
- 1/4 cup red bell bell pepper, diced
- 1/4 cup red onion, thinly sliced
- 2 tablespoons of tomato sauce
- 4 whole-wheat tortillas
- Guacamole (ripe avocado, lime juice, fresh cilantro, black pepper and salt)

Instructions:

1. In a bowl, mix the cooked quinoa with the black beans, corn, red bell bell pepper, red onion, and tomato sauce.
2. Heat whole-wheat tortillas in a lightly greased skillet.
3. Spread the quinoa and bean mixture over the tortillas.
4. Add the guacamole and roll the tortillas to form burritos.

49. Tomato and Basil Soup with Crostini

Ingredients for 2 persons:

- 6 ripe, diced tomatoes
- 1 onion, thinly sliced
- 2 cloves of garlic, minced
- 1 bunch of fresh basil
- 4 cups of vegetable broth
- 2 slices of whole wheat bread
- 2 tablespoons of extra virgin olive oil
- Sea salt and black pepper to taste

1. In a pot, sauté the onion and garlic in olive oil until tender.
2. Add diced tomatoes and fresh basil and cook for a few minutes.
3. Pour in the vegetable broth and bring to a boil. Reduce to medium-low heat and simmer for about 20 minutes.
4. In the meantime, toast the slices of whole wheat bread and spread them with a little olive oil.
5. Serve the tomato and basil soup with the bread croutons.

50. Salmon Salad with Avocado and Walnuts.

Ingredients for 2 persons:

- o 2 salmon fillets, cooked and filleted
- o 1 ripe avocado, sliced
- o 1/4 cup walnuts, coarsely chopped
- o 4 cups of mixed lettuce
- o 2 tablespoons of extra virgin olive oil
- o Juice of 1 lemon
- o Sea salt and black pepper to taste

Instructions:

1. In a bowl, mix the frayed salmon with sliced avocado, chopped walnuts, and mixed lettuce.
2. Prepare a vinaigrette with the olive oil, lemon juice, salt and pepper.
3. Dress the salad with the vinaigrette and serve.

51. Risotto with Porcini Mushrooms and Spinach

Ingredients for 2 persons:

- o 1 cup of Arborio rice
- o 1/2 onion, thinly sliced
- o 1 cup fresh or dried porcini mushrooms, sliced
- o 2 handfuls of fresh spinach
- o 1/4 cup of dry white wine
- o 4 cups of vegetable broth
- o 2 tablespoons of extra virgin olive oil
- o 2 tablespoons of grated parmesan cheese (optional)
- o Sea salt and black pepper to taste

Instructions:

1. Heat the vegetable broth in a pot and keep it hot.
2. In a frying pan, sauté the onion in olive oil until transparent.
3. Add porcini mushrooms and cook until golden brown.
4. Add the rice and lightly toast it.
5. Deglaze with white wine and let it evaporate.
6. Gradually add the hot broth, one ladleful at a time, stirring occasionally, until the risotto is creamy and the rice is cooked al dente.
7. Add fresh spinach and stir until wilted.
8. If desired, add grated Parmesan cheese and season with salt and pepper to taste.

52. Grilled Chicken Wraps with Vegetables and Hummus.

Ingredients for 2 persons:

- o 2 chicken breasts, marinated in olive oil, lemon juice, garlic, salt and pepper and then grilled
- o 4 whole wheat tortillas
- o Hummus (see recipe in previous subchapter)
- o 1 yellow bell pepper, cut into strips
- o 1 zucchini, thinly sliced
- o 1 carrot, thinly sliced
- o Mixed salad

Instructions:

1. Heat the whole-wheat tortillas in a lightly greased skillet.
2. Spread the hummus on the tortillas.
3. Add grilled chicken breasts, bell bell pepper strips, zucchini and carrot slices, and mixed salad.
4. Roll the tortillas to form wraps and serve.

53. Quinoa and Chickpea Meatballs with Tomato Sauce.

Ingredients for 2 persons:

- o 1 cup of cooked quinoa
- o 1 can of chickpeas, rinsed and drained
- o 1/4 cup red onion, thinly sliced
- o 2 cloves of garlic, minced
- o 1/4 cup chopped fresh parsley
- o 1 tablespoon of chickpea flour (or wheat flour)
- o Sea salt and black pepper to taste
- o Tomato sauce (tomato sauce, garlic, basil, salt and pepper)

Instructions:

1. In a food processor, blend the chickpeas with the garlic, parsley, and chickpea flour until smooth.
2. Transfer the mixture to a bowl and add the cooked quinoa and red onion. Stir well.
3. Form patties with the mixture and cook them in a lightly greased pan until golden brown.
4. Meanwhile, prepare the tomato sauce by cooking the tomato sauce with garlic, basil, salt and pepper.
5. Serve the quinoa and chickpea meatballs with the tomato sauce.

54. Mediterranean Couscous Salad

Ingredients for 2 persons:

- o 1 cup precooked couscous
- o 1/2 cucumber, diced
- o 1/2 red bell pepper, diced
- o 1/4 cup cherry tomatoes, cut in half
- o 1/4 cup black olives, pitted and sliced
- o 1/4 cup feta cheese, crumbled
- o 2 tablespoons of extra virgin olive oil
- o Juice of 1 lemon
- o Chopped fresh mint
- o Sea salt and black pepper to taste

Instructions:

1. Prepare the precooked couscous according to the instructions on the package.
2. In a bowl, mix the couscous with the cucumber, red bell pepper, cherry tomatoes, black olives, and feta.
3. Prepare a vinaigrette with the olive oil, lemon juice, salt and pepper.
4. Dress the couscous salad with the vinaigrette and sprinkle with chopped fresh mint.

55. Chickpea and Spinach Curry

Ingredients for 2 persons:

- o 1 can of chickpeas, rinsed and drained
- o 2 handfuls of fresh spinach
- o 1 onion, thinly sliced
- o 2 cloves of garlic, minced
- o 1 red bell pepper, diced
- o 1 tablespoon curry powder
- o 1 can of coconut milk
- o 2 tablespoons of extra virgin olive oil
- o Sea salt and black pepper to taste

Instructions:

1. Heat olive oil in a skillet and sauté the onion and garlic until tender.

2. Add the red bell pepper and cook until soft.
3. Add the chickpeas and curry powder and mix well.
4. Pour in the coconut milk and cook over medium-low heat for a few minutes.
5. Add fresh spinach and cook until wilted.
6. Season with salt and pepper to taste and serve the chickpea and spinach curry with basmati rice.

56. Baked Salmon with Asparagus

Ingredients for 2 persons:

- 2 salmon fillets
- 1 bunch of asparagus, chopped
- 2 tablespoons of extra virgin olive oil
- 1 clove of garlic, minced
- Juice of 1 lemon
- 1 tablespoon chopped fresh thyme
- Sea salt and black pepper to taste

Instructions:

1. Prepare a marinade with olive oil, garlic, lemon juice, thyme, salt and pepper.
2. Marinate the salmon fillets in the marinade for at least 30 minutes.
3. Preheat the oven to 375°F (about 190°C).
4. Arrange the salmon fillets and asparagus on a baking sheet lined with baking paper.
5. Bake for about 15 to 20 minutes, or until the salmon is cooked and the asparagus is tender.

57. Chicken Pita with Tzatziki Sauce

Ingredients for 2 persons:

- 2 whole-grain pita bread
- 2 chicken breasts, grilled and cut into strips
- 1 cucumber, thinly sliced
- 1 tomato, diced
- 1/4 cup red onion, thinly sliced
- Lettuce leaves
- Tzatziki sauce (Greek yogurt, grated cucumber, garlic, lemon juice, fresh mint, salt and pepper)

Instructions:

1. Heat whole-wheat pita bread in a lightly greased skillet.
2. Fill the pita with the grilled chicken strips, cucumber slices, tomato cubes, red onion, and lettuce leaves.
3. Add tzatziki sauce and serve chicken pita with tzatziki sauce as a light and tasty lunch.

58. Red Lentil Soup with Ginger.

Ingredients for 2 persons:

- 1 cup of red lentils
- 1 onion, thinly sliced
- 2 cloves of garlic, minced
- 1 tablespoon fresh grated ginger
- 1 carrot, diced
- 1 potato, diced
- 1 liter of vegetable broth
- 2 tablespoons of extra virgin olive oil
- Chopped fresh coriander
- Sea salt and black pepper to taste

Instructions:

1. Heat olive oil in a pot and sauté the onion and garlic until tender.
2. Add fresh grated ginger and cook for one minute.
3. Add the red lentils, carrot, and potato and mix well.
4. Pour in the vegetable broth and bring to a boil. Reduce to medium-low heat and simmer until the lentils and vegetables are soft.
5. Season with salt and pepper to taste and serve the red lentil soup with fresh chopped cilantro.

59. Chicken Salad with Avocado and Almonds.

Ingredients for 2 persons:

- 2 chicken breasts, cooked and cut into strips
- 1 ripe avocado, sliced
- 1/4 cup toasted almonds, coarsely chopped
- 4 cups of mixed lettuce
- 2 tablespoons of extra virgin olive oil
- Juice of 1 lemon
- Sea salt and black pepper to taste

Instructions:

1. In a bowl, mix cooked chicken with sliced avocado, chopped almonds, and mixed lettuce.
2. Prepare a vinaigrette with the olive oil, lemon juice, salt and pepper.
3. Dress the chicken salad with the vinaigrette and serve.

60. Vegetable Frittata with Spinach and Dried Tomatoes.

Ingredients for 2 persons:

- 6 eggs
- 2 handfuls of fresh spinach
- 1/4 cup sun-dried tomatoes, cut into strips
- 1/4 cup red onion, thinly sliced
- 2 tablespoons of extra virgin olive oil
- 2 tablespoons feta cheese, crumbled (optional)
- Sea salt and black pepper to taste

Instructions:

1. Heat olive oil in a skillet and sauté the red onion until tender.
2. Add fresh spinach and cook until wilted.

3. In a bowl, beat the eggs with salt and pepper.
4. Pour the eggs into the pan with the spinach and onion.
5. Add the sun-dried tomatoes and feta cheese, if desired.
6. Cook over medium-low heat until the omelet is cooked and golden brown.
7. Cut into wedges and serve the vegetable frittata with spinach and sun-dried tomatoes.

Addendum Sauces

1. Tzatziki sauce

Ingredients for 2 persons:

- 1 cup of Greek yogurt
- 1 cucumber, grated and well drained
- 1 clove of garlic, finely chopped
- Juice of half a lemon
- 1 tablespoon extra virgin olive oil
- 1 tablespoon fresh mint, chopped
- Sea salt and black pepper to taste

Instructions:

1. In a bowl, mix Greek yogurt with grated, drained cucumber.
2. Add the minced garlic, lemon juice, and extra virgin olive oil. Stir well.
3. Add chopped fresh mint and season with salt and pepper to taste. Stir again.
4. Cover the bowl and let it rest in the refrigerator for at least 30 minutes before serving.

2. Tomato Sauce

Ingredients for 2 persons:

- 1 can of peeled tomatoes
- 2 cloves of garlic, finely chopped
- 1 onion, thinly sliced

- o 2 tablespoons of extra virgin olive oil
- o 1 tablespoon chopped fresh basil
- o Sea salt and black pepper to taste

Instructions:

1. Heat olive oil in a pot and sauté the garlic and onion until tender.
2. Add the whole peeled tomatoes and mash them lightly with a fork.
3. Cook over medium-low heat for about 20 minutes, until the sauce thickens slightly.
4. Add chopped fresh basil and season with salt and pepper to taste. Stir well.
5. Let the tomato sauce cool before using it as a condiment for your recipes.

3. Guacamole

Ingredients for 2 persons:

- o 2 ripe avocados
- o Juice of 1 lime
- o 1 clove of garlic, finely chopped
- o 1/4 red onion, thinly sliced
- o 1 small tomato, diced
- o 1 tablespoon fresh cilantro, chopped
- o Sea salt and black pepper to taste

Instructions:

1. Peel the avocados, remove the pit and mash the pulp with a fork in a bowl.
2. Add the lime juice and stir well to prevent the avocado from blackening.
3. Add the minced garlic, red onion, tomato, and fresh cilantro to the avocado. Stir gently to combine the ingredients.
4. Season with salt and pepper to taste, adjusting the flavor according to your preference.
5. Cover the bowl with plastic wrap on top of the guacamole to prevent oxidation. Store in the refrigerator until ready to serve.

4: Light and tasty dinners

61. Mediterranean Quinoa and Chickpea Salad.

Ingredients for 2 persons:

- o 1 cup of cooked quinoa
- o 1 can of chickpeas, rinsed and drained
- o 1 cucumber, diced
- o 1 tomato, diced
- o 1/4 cup black olives, pitted and sliced
- o 2 tablespoons feta cheese, crumbled
- o 2 tablespoons of extra virgin olive oil
- o Juice of 1 lemon
- o Dried oregano
- o Sea salt and black pepper to taste

Instructions:

1. In a bowl, mix the cooked quinoa with the chickpeas, cucumber, tomato, and black olives.
2. Add feta cheese and season with olive oil, lemon juice, oregano, salt and pepper. Stir well.
3. Let it sit for a few minutes for the flavors to meld and serve this fresh and tasty Mediterranean quinoa and chickpea salad.

62. Chicken Curry with Vegetables

Ingredients for 2 persons:

- o 2 chicken breasts, cut into cubes
- o 1 zucchini, diced
- o 1 red bell pepper, diced
- o 1 onion, thinly sliced
- o 1 can of coconut milk
- o 2 tablespoons of extra virgin olive oil
- o 1 tablespoon curry powder
- o 1 tablespoon fresh cilantro, chopped
- o Sea salt and black pepper to taste

Instructions:

1. Heat olive oil in a frying pan and brown the onion until transparent.
2. Add the chicken cubes and cook them until golden brown and cooked through.
3. Add the zucchini and red bell pepper and continue cooking for a few minutes.
4. Pour in the coconut milk and mix well. Add curry powder, salt and pepper.
5. Let cook over medium-low heat until the vegetables are tender and the sauce has thickened slightly.
6. Serve the chicken curry with vegetables, sprinkled with fresh chopped cilantro.

63. Grilled Shrimp with Mango and Avocado Sauce.

Ingredients for 2 persons:

- 10.6 ounces of shrimp, shelled and cleaned
- 1 tablespoon extra virgin olive oil
- Juice of 1 lime
- 1 clove of garlic, minced
- 1 ripe mango, cut into cubes
- 1 ripe avocado, cut into cubes
- 1 red chili pepper, finely chopped (optional for spicy touch)
- Chopped fresh parsley
- Sea salt and black pepper to taste

Instructions:

1. In a bowl, mix shrimp with olive oil, lime juice, garlic, salt, and pepper.
2. Heat a grill and cook the shrimp until cooked and lightly browned.
3. In another bowl, mix mango with avocado, chili (if desired) and parsley. Season with salt and pepper.
4. Serve the grilled shrimp accompanied by the mango and avocado salsa.

64. Red Lentil and Spinach Soup.

Ingredients for 2 persons:

- 1 cup of red lentils
- 1 onion, thinly sliced
- 2 carrots, cut into rounds
- 2 stalks of celery, diced
- 2 cloves of garlic, minced
- 4 cups of vegetable broth
- 2 cups of fresh spinach
- 1 tablespoon extra virgin olive oil
- 1 teaspoon turmeric powder
- 1 teaspoon cumin powder
- Sea salt and black pepper to taste

Instructions:

1. Heat olive oil in a saucepan and brown the onion until transparent.
2. Add the carrots, celery, and garlic, and continue cooking for a few minutes.
3. Add the red lentils, turmeric, cumin, salt and pepper, and mix well.
4. Pour in the vegetable broth and bring to a boil. Then reduce the heat and cook over medium heat for about 15 to 20 minutes or until the lentils are tender.
5. Add fresh spinach and let it wilt in the soup.
6. Serve red lentil and spinach soup as a light and healthy main dish.

65. Vegetable Frittata with Smoked Salmon

Ingredients for 2 persons:

- 4 eggs
- 1 zucchini, diced
- 1 red bell pepper, diced
- 1 onion, thinly sliced
- ounces of smoked salmon, cut into strips
- 1 tablespoon of extra virgin olive oil
- Chopped fresh parsley

o Sea salt and black pepper to taste

Instructions:

1. Heat olive oil in a frying pan and brown the onion until transparent.
2. Add the zucchini and red bell pepper and cook until the vegetables are tender.
3. In a bowl, beat eggs with salt, pepper and chopped parsley.
4. Pour the beaten eggs into the pan with the vegetables and add the smoked salmon strips.
5. Cook the omelet over medium-low heat until it is well set and golden brown.
6. Serve vegetable frittata with smoked salmon as a light but tasty dinner.

66. Sesame Chicken Bowl with Grilled Vegetables.

Ingredients for 2 persons:

o 2 chicken breasts, cooked and cut into strips
o 1 cup of cooked brown rice
o 1 zucchini, cut into strips and grilled
o 1 yellow bell pepper, cut into strips and grilled
o 1 carrot, cut into strips and grilled
o 2 tablespoons of toasted sesame seeds
o 2 tablespoons of low-sodium soy sauce
o 1 tablespoon of sesame oil
o 1 tablespoon of rice vinegar
o 1 teaspoon fresh ginger, grated
o 1 teaspoon garlic, minced
o 1 green onion, thinly sliced
o Fresh red chili pepper, thinly sliced (optional for spicy touch)
o Chopped fresh parsley
o Sea salt and black pepper to taste

Instructions:

1. In a bowl, mix the chicken with the soy sauce, sesame oil, rice vinegar, ginger, and garlic.
2. Heat the marinated chicken in a skillet until well heated.
3. In 2 bowls, spread the cooked brown rice and lay the grilled vegetables on top of it.
4. Spread the sesame chicken over the grilled vegetables and sprinkle with toasted sesame seeds.
5. Garnish with green onion, sliced red pepper (if desired) and fresh parsley.
6. Serve the sesame chicken bowl with grilled vegetables for a healthy and tasty dinner.

67. Grilled Salmon with Asparagus and Sweet Potatoes.

Ingredients for 2 persons:

o 2 salmon fillets
o 1 bunch of asparagus, lightly peeled
o 1 large sweet potato, diced
o 2 tablespoons of extra virgin olive oil
o 1 clove of garlic, minced
o Juice of 1/2 lemon
o Chopped fresh parsley
o Sea salt and black pepper to taste

Instructions:

1. In a bowl, mix asparagus and sweet potatoes with olive oil, garlic, salt and pepper.
2. Heat a grill and cook asparagus and sweet potatoes until tender and lightly browned.
3. Brush the salmon fillets with olive oil and grill them until cooked and lightly browned.
4. Serve the grilled salmon accompanied by the asparagus and sweet potatoes. Drizzle with lemon juice and sprinkle with chopped fresh parsley.

68. Chicken with Sun-Dried Tomatoes and Spinach.

Ingredients for 2 persons:

- 2 chicken breasts
- 1 cup sun-dried tomatoes soaked in hot water
- 2 handfuls of fresh spinach
- 2 tablespoons of extra virgin olive oil
- 2 tablespoons balsamic vinegar
- 1 tablespoon dried oregano
- 1 clove of garlic, minced
- Sea salt and black pepper to taste

Instructions:

1. Heat olive oil in a frying pan and sauté garlic until lightly browned.
2. Add the chicken breasts and cook them until cooked and browned.
3. Add the sun-dried tomatoes, spinach and balsamic vinegar. Stir well.
4. Sprinkle with dried oregano, salt and pepper.
5. Let it cook until the spinach is wilted and the flavors are well blended.
6. Serve the chicken with sun-dried tomatoes and spinach for a tasty and healthy dinner.

69. Fish Taco with Guacamole

Ingredients for 2 persons:

- 10.6 ounces of white fish fillets (such as tilapia or cod)
- 4 corn or whole wheat tortillas
- 1 ripe avocado
- Juice of 1 lime
- 1/4 red onion, finely chopped
- 1 tomato, diced
- Chopped fresh coriander
- Fresh red chili pepper, thinly sliced (optional for spicy touch)

- Sea salt and black pepper to taste

Instructions:

1. Heat a nonstick skillet and cook the fish fillets until they are cooked and easily crumbled with a fork.
2. In a bowl, mash the avocado with the lime juice, red onion, tomato, cilantro, chili (if desired), salt and pepper.
3. Heat tortillas in another skillet until hot and slightly crispy.
4. Fill each tortilla with the cooked fish and a spoonful of guacamole.
5. Serve fish tacos with guacamole as a light and tasty dinner.

70. Paprika Chicken Chunks with Quinoa and Broccoli.

Ingredients for 2 persons:

- 2 chicken breasts, cut into bite-sized pieces
- 1 cup of cooked quinoa
- 1 bunch of broccoli, cut into florets
- 2 tablespoons of extra virgin olive oil
- 1 tablespoon paprika
- 1 teaspoon garlic powder
- 1 teaspoon onion powder
- Sea salt and black pepper to taste

Instructions:

1. Heat olive oil in a skillet and brown the chicken nuggets until golden brown and cooked through.
2. Add paprika, garlic powder, onion powder, salt and pepper. Stir well.
3. Steam the broccoli until tender but crisp.
4. On 2 plates, spread the cooked quinoa and lay the paprika chicken bites on top of it.
5. Garnish with steamed broccoli.

6. Serve paprika chicken bites with quinoa and broccoli for a complete and nutritious dinner.

71. Eggplant Roulades with Ricotta and Tomatoes.

Ingredients for 2 persons:

o 2 long eggplants, thinly sliced
o 1 cup of cottage cheese
o 1 cup of tomato puree
o 1 clove of garlic, minced
o 1 bunch of fresh basil, chopped
o 2 tablespoons of extra virgin olive oil
o Sea salt and black pepper to taste

Instructions:

1. Heat olive oil in a frying pan and sauté garlic until lightly browned.
2. Add the tomato puree and let it cook over medium-low heat for a few minutes.
3. In a bowl, mix ricotta cheese with chopped basil, salt and pepper.
4. Take a slice of eggplant and spread a small amount of ricotta cheese in the center. Roll up the slice and place it in a lightly greased baking dish.
5. Repeat the process with the remaining eggplant slices and the remaining ricotta.
6. Pour the tomato sauce over the top of the eggplant rolls and bake in a 350°F (180°C) oven for about 20 minutes or until the eggplant is soft and the cheese is melted.
7. Serve eggplant rolls with ricotta and tomatoes as a tasty vegetarian dinner.

72. Salmon and Avocado Salad

o Ingredients for 2 persons:
o 2 cooked and crumbled salmon fillets
o 1 ripe avocado, cut into cubes
o 1 cucumber, diced
o 1 tomato, diced

o 2 tablespoons of extra virgin olive oil
o Juice of 1 lemon
o Chopped fresh parsley
o Sea salt and black pepper to taste

Instructions:

1. In a bowl, mix the crumbled salmon with the avocado, cucumber and tomato.
2. Season with olive oil, lemon juice, salt and pepper.
3. Sprinkle with fresh chopped parsley.
4. Serve salmon and avocado salad as a light and tasty dinner.

73. Lentil and Vegetable Soup.

Ingredients for 2 persons:

o 1 cup of green lentils
o 2 carrots, cut into rounds
o 2 stalks of celery, diced
o 1 onion, thinly sliced
o 2 cloves of garlic, minced
o 4 cups of vegetable broth
o 1 bunch of fresh parsley, chopped
o 1 tablespoon extra virgin olive oil
o Sea salt and black pepper to taste

Instructions:

1. Heat olive oil in a pan and sauté the onion and garlic until golden brown.
2. Add the carrots and celery and continue cooking for a few minutes.
3. Add the green lentils and vegetable broth. Bring to a boil, then reduce the heat and cook over medium heat for about 20-25 minutes or until the lentils are tender.
4. Season with salt and pepper to taste and sprinkle with fresh chopped parsley.
5. Serve lentil and vegetable soup for a nutritious, warming dinner.

74. Grilled Tofu with Peanut and Broccoli Sauce.

Ingredients for 2 persons:

- 1 cup tofu, cut into cubes
- 1 bunch of broccoli, cut into florets and steamed
- 2 tablespoons of peanut sauce
- 2 tablespoons of low-sodium soy sauce
- 1 tablespoon of sesame oil
- 1 teaspoon fresh ginger, grated
- 1 teaspoon garlic, minced
- 1 tablespoon fresh chopped parsley
- Fresh red chili pepper, thinly sliced (optional for spicy touch)

Sea salt and black pepper to taste

Instructions:

1. In a bowl, mix the peanut sauce, soy sauce, sesame oil, ginger and garlic.
2. Add the tofu cubes to the marinade and let it sit for at least 15 to 20 minutes.
3. Heat a grill and cook the tofu until golden brown and crispy.
4. In 2 plates, spread the steamed broccoli and lay the grilled tofu on top of them.
5. Sprinkle with fresh chopped parsley and sliced red chili pepper (if desired).
6. Serve grilled tofu with peanut sauce and broccoli for a tasty vegan dinner.

75. Spinach and Mushroom Frittata.

Ingredients for 2 persons:

- 4 eggs
- 1 cup of fresh spinach
- ounces of button mushrooms, sliced
- 1 onion, thinly sliced
- 2 tablespoons of extra virgin olive oil
- 2 tablespoons of milk (choice of cow's milk or vegetable milk)
- 1 tablespoon of grated cheese (your choice of parmesan or pecorino)
- Chopped fresh parsley
- Sea salt and black pepper to taste

Instructions:

1. Heat olive oil in a frying pan and brown the onion until transparent.
2. Add the champignon mushrooms and continue cooking until golden brown and cooked through.
3. In a bowl, beat eggs with milk, grated cheese, chopped parsley, salt and pepper.
4. Add fresh spinach to the pan and cook until wilted.
5. Pour the egg mixture over the skillet with the spinach and mushrooms.
6. Cook the omelet over medium-low heat until it is well set and golden brown.
7. Serve spinach and mushroom frittata as a light and tasty dinner.

76. Teriyaki Salmon with Grilled Vegetables.

Ingredients for 2 persons:

- 2 salmon fillets
- 1 cup broccoli, floreted and grilled
- 1 red bell pepper, cut into strips and grilled
- 1 carrot, cut into strips and grilled
- 2 tablespoons teriyaki sauce
- 1 tablespoon extra virgin olive oil
- 1 tablespoon of lemon juice
- 1 tablespoon of honey (optional)
- Chopped fresh parsley
- Sea salt and black pepper to taste

Instructions:

1. In a bowl, mix the teriyaki sauce, olive oil, lemon juice, and honey (if desired).
2. Brush the salmon with the marinade and let it rest for at least 15 minutes.

3. Heat a grill and cook the salmon until cooked and lightly browned.
4. Spread the grilled broccoli, bell bell pepper, and carrot among 2 plates.
5. Lay the teriyaki salmon on top of the grilled vegetables.
6. Sprinkle with fresh chopped parsley and salt and pepper to taste.
7. Serve teriyaki salmon with grilled vegetables for a delicious and nutritious dinner.

77. Curried Quinoa with Chickpeas and Vegetables.

Ingredients for 2 persons:

- 1 cup of cooked quinoa
- 1 can of chickpeas, rinsed and drained
- 1 zucchini, diced and steamed
- 1 red bell pepper, diced and steamed
- 1 onion, thinly sliced
- 2 tablespoons of extra virgin olive oil
- 2 tablespoons of coconut milk
- 1 teaspoon curry powder
- Chopped fresh parsley
- Sea salt and black pepper to taste

Instructions:

1. Heat olive oil in a frying pan and brown the onion until transparent.
2. Add the steamed chickpeas, zucchini, and red bell pepper and mix well.
3. Add the cooked quinoa and stir again.
4. Pour in the coconut milk and curry powder. Stir until the ingredients are well blended.
5. Let cook over medium-low heat until all ingredients are well heated.
6. Serve curried quinoa with chickpeas and vegetables as a tasty vegan dinner.

78. Cous Cous and Lemon Chicken Salad.

Ingredients for 2 persons:

- 2 chicken breasts, cooked and cut into strips
- 1 cup of cooked couscous
- 1 cucumber, diced
- 1 tomato, diced
- 1/4 red onion, thinly sliced
- 2 tablespoons of extra virgin olive oil
- Juice of 1 lemon
- Chopped fresh parsley
- Sea salt and black pepper to taste

Instructions:

1. In a bowl, mix the cooked chicken with the cous cous, cucumber, tomato, and red onion.
2. Season with olive oil, lemon juice, chopped fresh parsley, salt and pepper.
3. Stir well and let stand for a few minutes for the flavors to blend.
4. Serve couscous salad and lemon chicken as a light and tasty dinner.

79. Whole wheat pasta with arugula pesto and cherry tomatoes

Ingredients for 2 persons:

- 3 + 2/3 cups of whole wheat pasta
- 2 cups of fresh arugula
- 1/2 cup walnuts
- 1/2 cup of grated parmesan cheese
- 1 clove of garlic
- 1 cup cherry tomatoes, cut in half
- 2 tablespoons of extra virgin olive oil
- Sea salt and black pepper to taste

Instructions:

1. Cook whole wheat pasta in salted water following the instructions on the package.
2. Meanwhile, prepare the arugula pesto. In a blender, blend the arugula, walnuts, Parmesan cheese, garlic, olive oil, salt, and pepper until smooth.
3. Drain the pasta and pour it into a bowl.
4. Season the pasta with the arugula pesto and mix well.
5. Add the halved cherry tomatoes and stir again.
6. Serve whole wheat pasta with arugula pesto and cherry tomatoes for a simple but delicious dinner.

80. Sesame Tofu with Broccoli and Rice

Ingredients for 2 persons:

- 1 cup tofu, cut into cubes
- 1 bunch of broccoli, cut into florets and steamed
- 1 cup of cooked brown rice
- 2 tablespoons of low-sodium soy sauce
- 1 tablespoon of sesame oil
- 1 tablespoon of toasted sesame seeds
- Sea salt and black pepper to taste

Instructions:

1. Heat the sesame oil in a frying pan and add the tofu cubes. Cook the tofu until golden brown and crispy.
2. Add the steamed broccoli to the pan with the tofu and mix well.
3. Pour the soy sauce over the tofu and broccoli and stir again.
4. In 2 plates, spread the cooked brown rice and lay the sesame tofu and broccoli on top of it.
5. Sprinkle with toasted sesame seeds, salt and pepper to taste.
6. Serve sesame tofu with broccoli and rice for a tasty vegan dinner.

81. Quinoa Salad with Shrimp and Avocado.

Ingredients for 2 persons:

- 1 cup of cooked quinoa
- 7 ounces of shrimp, shelled and cleaned
- 1 ripe avocado, cut into cubes
- 1 tomato, diced
- 2 tablespoons of extra virgin olive oil
- Juice of 1 lemon
- Chopped fresh parsley
- Sea salt and black pepper to taste

Instructions:

1. In a bowl, mix shrimp with olive oil, lemon juice, chopped parsley, salt and pepper.
2. Heat a skillet and cook the shrimp until cooked and lightly browned.
3. In another bowl, mix the cooked quinoa with the avocado, tomato, and cooked shrimp.
4. Season with olive oil, lemon juice, chopped parsley, salt and pepper.
5. Serve quinoa salad with shrimp and avocado as a light and tasty dinner.

82. Salmon with Dill and Zucchini Sauce.

Ingredients for 2 persons:

- 2 salmon fillets
- 2 zucchini, cut into rounds and steamed
- 1 onion, thinly sliced
- 2 tablespoons of extra virgin olive oil
- 1 tablespoon of mustard
- 1 tablespoon of honey
- Juice of 1/2 lemon
- 1 tablespoon fresh dill, chopped
- Sea salt and black pepper to taste

1. Heat olive oil in a frying pan and brown the onion until transparent.
2. Add the salmon fillets and cook them until cooked and golden brown.
3. In a bowl, mix mustard, honey, lemon juice, dill, salt and pepper.
4. Pour the dill sauce over the salmon and let it sit for a few minutes for the flavors to meld.
5. Serve salmon with dill sauce accompanied by steamed zucchini for a tasty and nutritious dinner.

83. Zucchini and Lemon Risotto

Ingredients for 2 persons:

- 1 cup of Arborio or Carnaroli rice
- 2 zucchini, diced
- 1 onion, thinly sliced
- 2 tablespoons of extra virgin olive oil
- 1/2 cup of dry white wine
- 3 cups of vegetable broth
- Grated zest of 1 lemon
- Juice of 1 lemon
- 1 tablespoon fresh chopped parsley
- Sea salt and black pepper to taste

Instructions:

1. Heat olive oil in a saucepan and brown the onion until transparent.
2. Add zucchini and cook until tender.
3. Add the rice and toast it for a few minutes.
4. Pour in the white wine and let the alcohol evaporate.
5. Add the vegetable broth, one ladleful at a time, stirring occasionally and waiting for it to be absorbed before adding more. Continue until the rice is cooked al dente and the mixture is creamy.
6. Add grated zest and lemon juice. Stir well.

7. Season with salt, pepper and chopped parsley.
8. Serve zucchini and lemon risotto as a fine and delicious dinner.

84. Chicken with Mango Sauce and Basmati Rice.

Ingredients for 2 persons:

- 2 chicken breasts
- 1 cup of cooked basmati rice
- 1 ripe mango, peeled and diced
- 1 red chili pepper, seedless and thinly sliced
- 1 clove of garlic, minced
- 2 tablespoons of extra virgin olive oil
- 2 tablespoons apple cider vinegar
- Chopped fresh parsley
- Sea salt and black pepper to taste

Instructions:

1. Heat the olive oil in a frying pan and sauté the garlic and chili until golden brown.
2. Add the chicken breasts and cook them until cooked and browned.
3. In a bowl, mix the mango with the apple cider vinegar.
4. In 2 plates, spread the cooked basmati rice and lay the chicken on top of it.
5. Pour the mango sauce over the chicken and rice.
6. Sprinkle with fresh chopped parsley, salt and pepper to taste.
7. Serve the chicken with mango salsa and basmati rice for an exotic and tasty dinner.

85. Chickpea and Arugula Salad

Ingredients for 2 persons:

- 2 cups of cooked chickpeas
- 2 cups of fresh arugula

- 1 yellow bell pepper, diced
- 1/4 red onion, thinly sliced
- 1/2 cucumber, diced
- 2 tablespoons of extra virgin olive oil
- Juice of 1 lemon
- Chopped fresh parsley
- Sea salt and black pepper to taste

Instructions:

1. In a bowl, mix the chickpeas with the arugula, yellow bell pepper, red onion, and cucumber.
2. Season with olive oil, lemon juice, chopped fresh parsley, salt and pepper.
3. Stir well and let stand for a few minutes for the flavors to blend.
4. Serve chickpea and arugula salad as a light and tasty dinner.

86. Chicken with Homemade Barbecue Sauce and Baked Sweet Potatoes.

Ingredients for 2 persons:

- 2 chicken breasts
- 2 large sweet potatoes, diced
- 2 tablespoons of extra virgin olive oil
- 1/4 cup of tomato sauce
- 2 tablespoons Worcestershire sauce (check for gluten-free if needed)
- 2 tablespoons apple cider vinegar
- 1 tablespoon of honey
- 1 teaspoon of mustard
- 1/2 teaspoon garlic powder
- 1/2 teaspoon onion powder
- 1/2 teaspoon paprika
- Sea salt and black pepper to taste

Instructions:

1. Heat the oven to 200°C (390°F).
2. In a bowl, mix tomato sauce, Worcestershire sauce, apple cider vinegar, honey, mustard, garlic powder, onion powder, paprika, salt and pepper.

3. In another bowl, mix the sweet potato cubes with a tablespoon of olive oil and a sprinkle of salt.
4. Place the sweet potato cubes on a baking sheet lined with baking paper and bake in the oven for about 25 to 30 minutes or until soft and golden brown.
5. Meanwhile, heat a skillet with a tablespoon of olive oil and cook the chicken breasts until they are cooked through and golden brown on both sides.
6. Pour the homemade barbecue sauce over the skillet with the chicken and season for a few minutes until the chicken is well coated with the sauce.
7. Serve the chicken with barbecue sauce and baked sweet potatoes for a tasty, home-cooked dinner.

87. Pasta with Basil Pesto and Cherry Tomatoes

Ingredients for 2 persons:

- 2 + 2/3 cups of pasta (such as spaghetti or penne)
- 1 bunch of fresh basil
- 1/2 cup walnuts
- 1/2 cup grated cheese (your choice of parmesan or pecorino)
- 1 cup cherry tomatoes, cut in half
- 2 tablespoons of extra virgin olive oil
- 1 clove of garlic
- Sea salt and black pepper to taste

Instructions:

1. Cook the pasta in plenty of salted water following the instructions on the package.
2. Meanwhile, prepare the basil pesto. In a blender, blend basil, walnuts, grated cheese, garlic, olive oil, salt, and pepper until smooth.
3. Drain the pasta al dente and pour it into a bowl.

4. Season the pasta with the basil pesto and mix well.
5. Add the halved cherry tomatoes and stir again.
6. Serve pasta with basil pesto and cherry tomatoes as a simple but delicious dinner.

88. Chicken Cacciatora with Polenta

Ingredients for 2 persons:

- o 2 chicken thighs with over-thighs
- o 1 cup of tomato puree
- o 1/2 cup of red wine
- o 1 onion, thinly sliced
- o 2 cloves of garlic, minced
- o 2 tablespoons of extra virgin olive oil
- o 1 sprig of fresh rosemary
- o 1 sprig of fresh thyme
- o Sea salt and black pepper to taste
- o 1 cup cornmeal for polenta
- o 4 cups of water
- o 1/2 cup grated cheese (your choice of parmesan or pecorino)
- o 2 tablespoons of butter

Instructions:

1. Heat olive oil in a pan and sauté the onion and garlic until golden brown.
2. Add the chicken thighs and cook them until golden brown on all sides.
3. Pour the red wine into the pot and let the alcohol evaporate.
4. Add the tomato puree, rosemary, thyme, salt and pepper. Cover with a lid and cook on low heat for about 30-40 minutes or until the chicken is tender and well cooked.
5. Meanwhile, prepare the polenta. In a pot, bring water to a boil and add a pinch of salt.
6. Sprinkle the cornmeal into the pot, stirring constantly to avoid lumps.
7. Continue to stir the polenta over medium-low heat until it becomes thick and creamy.

8. Remove from heat and stir in grated cheese and butter until well blended.
9. Serve chicken cacciatore with polenta as a rustic and tasty dinner.

89. Rice and Tuna Salad

Ingredients for 2 persons:

- o 1 cup of cooked basmati rice
- o 1 can of tuna drained and crumbled
- o 1/2 cup corn
- o 1/2 cup of peas
- o 1/4 red onion, thinly sliced
- o 1/4 yellow bell pepper, diced
- o 2 tablespoons of extra virgin olive oil
- o Juice of 1 lemon
- o Chopped fresh parsley
- o Sea salt and black pepper to taste

Instructions:

1. In a bowl, mix basmati rice with crumbled tuna, corn, peas, red onion, and yellow bell pepper.
2. Season with olive oil, lemon juice, chopped fresh parsley, salt and pepper.
3. Stir well and let stand for a few minutes for the flavors to blend.
4. Serve rice and tuna salad as a light and tasty dinner.

90. Gnocchi with Zucchini Pesto.

Ingredients for 2 persons:

- o ounces of fresh or dried dumplings
- o 2 zucchini, cut into rounds and steamed
- o 1/2 cup walnuts
- o 1/2 cup grated cheese (your choice of parmesan or pecorino)
- o 2 tablespoons of extra virgin olive oil
- o 1 clove of garlic
- o Chopped fresh parsley
- o Sea salt and black pepper to taste

Instructions:

1. Cook the gnocchi in plenty of salted water following the instructions on the package.
2. Meanwhile, prepare the zucchini pesto. In a blender, blend steamed zucchini, walnuts, grated cheese, garlic, olive oil, salt, and pepper until smooth.
3. Drain the gnocchi and pour them into a bowl.
4. Season the gnocchi with the zucchini pesto and mix well.
5. Serve gnocchi with zucchini pesto sprinkled with fresh chopped parsley for a delicious, vegetarian dinner.
6. Sure enough, here are the explanations for the preparations of the two sauces to be included in the "Sauces" addendum:

Addendum Sauces

Dill Sauce for Teriyaki Salmon

Ingredients:

- 1/4 cup of mayonnaise
- 1 tablespoon of mustard
- 1 tablespoon of lemon juice
- 1 tablespoon fresh chopped dill
- Salt and black pepper to taste

Instructions:

- In a bowl, mix the mayonnaise, mustard, and lemon juice until smooth.
- Add chopped fresh dill and mix well.
- Taste and adjust the salt and black pepper to suit your taste.
- The dill sauce is ready to be served with the teriyaki salmon and grilled vegetables.

Zucchini Pesto for Gnocchi

Ingredients:

- 2 medium zucchini, cut into rounds

- 1/4 cup roasted almonds
- 1/4 cup of grated cheese (your choice of parmesan or pecorino)
- 2 tablespoons of extra virgin olive oil
- 1 clove of garlic
- Chopped fresh parsley
- Sea salt and black pepper to taste

Instructions:

1. In a frying pan, heat a tablespoon of olive oil and add the zucchini.
2. Cook zucchini until tender and lightly browned.
3. In a blender, blend the cooked zucchini, toasted almonds, grated cheese, garlic, parsley, salt, and black pepper until smooth.
4. Add the second tablespoon of olive oil and stir again.
5. The zucchini pesto is ready to be tossed on the gnocchi.

5: Guilt-free desserts

91. Vanilla Coconut Chia Pudding.

Ingredients for 2 persons:

- 1/4 cup chia seeds
- 1 cup of coconut milk (no added sugar) or other vegetable milk
- 1 teaspoon honey or maple syrup
- 1/2 teaspoon vanilla extract
- Fresh fruit for garnish (strawberries, blueberries or raspberries are good)

Instructions:

1. In a bowl, mix chia seeds, coconut milk, honey or maple syrup, and vanilla extract.
2. Mix well and let stand for at least 15-20 minutes or until the mixture becomes gelatinous.
3. Pour the vanilla coconut chia pudding into two bowls.

4. Garnish with fresh fruit before serving.

92. Apple Cinnamon Muffins.

Ingredients for 2 persons:

- o 1 cup of whole wheat flour
- o 1 teaspoon baking powder
- o 1/4 teaspoon baking soda
- o 1/4 teaspoon salt
- o 1 teaspoon cinnamon powder
- o 1 egg
- o 1/4 cup honey or maple syrup
- o 1/4 cup coconut milk (no added sugar) or other vegetable milk
- o 1 large apple, peeled and grated
- o 1/4 cup chopped walnuts

Instructions:

1. Preheat the oven to 180°C (350°F) and line a muffin mold with paper cups.
2. In a bowl, mix the whole wheat flour, baking powder, baking soda, salt and cinnamon.
3. In another bowl, mix the egg, honey or maple syrup, coconut milk, and grated apple.
4. Combine the wet ingredients with the dry ingredients and mix until smooth.
5. Add chopped walnuts and mix gently.
6. Pour the batter into the paper cups in the muffin mold.
7. Bake for about 15 to 18 minutes or until muffins are golden brown and cooked inside.
8. Let cool before enjoying the delicious apple-cinnamon muffins.

93. Antioxidant Green Smoothie

Ingredients for 2 persons:

- o 1 cup of fresh spinach
- o 1 cup fresh kale
- o 1/2 ripe avocado

- o 1/2 banana
- o 1 cup of coconut water or other liquid of your choice (coconut milk, almond milk)
- o 1 tablespoon of chia seeds
- o 1 teaspoon honey or maple syrup (optional)

Instructions:

1. Place spinach, kale, avocado, banana, and coconut water in high-power blender.
2. Blend until smooth and creamy.
3. If you want a sweet touch, you can add a teaspoon of honey or maple syrup and blend again.
4. Pour the green smoothie into two glasses.
5. Sprinkle chia seeds on top before serving.

94. Fresh Fruit with Yogurt and Mint Sauce.

Ingredients for 2 persons:

- o 1 cup of fresh sliced strawberries
- o 1 cup of fresh blueberries
- o 1 cup of Greek yogurt (no added sugar) or coconut yogurt
- o 1 teaspoon honey or maple syrup
- o 1 teaspoon chopped fresh mint leaves

Instructions:

1. Arrange the strawberries and blueberries in two bowls.
2. In a small bowl, mix yogurt, honey or maple syrup and chopped mint.
3. Pour the yogurt sauce over the fresh fruit and stir gently before serving.

95. Banana Coconut Ice Cream

Ingredients for 2 persons:

- o 2 ripe frozen bananas
- o 1/4 cup coconut milk (no added sugar) or other vegetable milk

- 1/4 teaspoon vanilla extract
- Fresh fruit and grated coconut for garnish (optional)

Instructions:

1. Cut the frozen bananas into pieces and place them in a high-power blender.
2. Add the coconut milk and vanilla extract.
3. Blend until creamy and smooth.
4. Pour the banana-coconut ice cream into two bowls.
5. Garnish with fresh fruit and grated coconut, if desired.
6. Serve immediately to enjoy this delicious guilt-free ice cream dessert.

96. Avocado Mousse with Cocoa

Ingredients for 2 persons:

- 1 ripe avocado
- 1/4 cup coconut milk (no added sugar) or other vegetable milk
- 2 tablespoons of cocoa powder
- 1 teaspoon honey or maple syrup (optional)
- Fresh fruit for garnish (strawberries, raspberries or blueberries are good)

Instructions:

1. In a high-powered blender, blend the avocado, coconut milk, and cocoa powder until smooth and creamy.
2. If you want a sweet touch, you can add a teaspoon of honey or maple syrup and blend again.
3. Pour the cocoa avocado mousse into two bowls.
4. Garnish with fresh fruit before serving.

97. Oatmeal and Apple Muffins

Ingredients for 2 persons:

- 1 cup oatmeal (finely ground oats)
- 1 teaspoon baking powder
- 1/2 teaspoon cinnamon powder
- 1/4 teaspoon nutmeg
- 1/4 teaspoon salt
- 1/2 cup coconut milk (no added sugar) or other vegetable milk
- 1/4 cup honey or maple syrup
- 1 egg
- 1 large apple, peeled and grated
- 1/4 cup chopped walnuts

Instructions:

1. Preheat the oven to 180°C (350°F) and line a muffin mold with paper cups.
2. In a bowl, mix the oat flour, baking powder, cinnamon, nutmeg, and salt.
3. In another bowl, mix the coconut milk, honey or maple syrup and egg.
4. Combine the wet ingredients with the dry ingredients and mix until smooth.
5. Add the grated apple and chopped walnuts and mix gently.
6. Pour the batter into the paper cups in the muffin mold.
7. Bake for about 15 to 18 minutes or until muffins are golden brown and cooked inside.
8. Let cool before enjoying the delicious oatmeal and apple muffins.

98. Fruit and Yogurt Cups

Ingredients for 2 persons:

- 1 cup of fresh sliced strawberries
- 1 cup of fresh blueberries
- 1 cup of Greek yogurt (no added sugar) or coconut yogurt
- 1 teaspoon honey or maple syrup (optional)

- Chopped walnuts and grated coconut for garnish (optional)

Instructions:

1. Arrange the strawberries and blueberries in two glasses or bowls.
2. Pour the yogurt over the fresh fruit.
3. If you want a sweet touch, you can add a teaspoon of honey or maple syrup.
4. Garnish with chopped nuts and grated coconut, if desired.
5. Serve the fruit and yogurt cups as a light and refreshing dessert.

99. Banana and Chocolate Smoothie.

Ingredients for 2 persons:

- 2 ripe bananas
- 2 cups of almond milk (no added sugar) or other vegetable milk
- 2 tablespoons of cocoa powder
- 1 teaspoon honey or maple syrup (optional)
- Ice (optional)

Instructions:

1. Place bananas, almond milk, and cocoa powder in high-power blender.
2. Blend until smooth and creamy.
3. If you want a sweet touch, you can add a teaspoon of honey or maple syrup and blend again.
4. If you prefer a thicker smoothie, add some ice and blend again.
5. Pour the banana-chocolate smoothie into two glasses and enjoy immediately.

100. Coconut Mango Pudding

Ingredients for 2 persons:

- 1 cup of coconut milk (no added sugar) or other vegetable milk

- 1 cup diced fresh mango
- 2 tablespoons of chia seeds
- 1 teaspoon honey or maple syrup (optional)
- Fresh sliced mango and grated coconut for garnish (optional)

Instructions:

1. In a bowl, mix coconut milk and diced mango.
2. Add the chia seeds and mix well.
3. Cover the bowl with plastic wrap and refrigerate it for at least 2 hours or until the mixture becomes gelatinous.
4. If you want a sweet touch, you can add a teaspoon of honey or maple syrup and stir again.
5. Pour the coconut-mango pudding into two bowls and garnish with fresh mango slices and grated coconut, if desired.

101. Cup of Strawberries with Creamy Walnuts.

Ingredients for 2 persons:

- 2 cups of fresh strawberries cut in half
- 1 cup of soaked walnuts (soak them in water for at least 4 hours and drain before using)
- 1/2 cup of water
- 1 tablespoon honey or maple syrup (optional)

Instructions:

1. Place the soaked walnuts and water in a high-power blender.
2. Blend until smooth and homogeneous.
3. If you want a sweet touch, you can add a tablespoon of honey or maple syrup and blend again.
4. Arrange the halved strawberries in two bowls.

5. Pour the walnut cream over the strawberries before serving.

102. Almond Flour Cookies.

Ingredients for 2 persons:

- o 1 cup of almond flour
- o 1/4 teaspoon baking soda
- o 1/4 teaspoon salt
- o 1 tablespoon coconut oil (melted)
- o 1 tablespoon honey or maple syrup
- o 1 egg
- o 1 teaspoon vanilla extract
- o Whole almonds for garnish (optional)

Instructions:

1. Preheat the oven to 180°C (350°F) and line a baking sheet with baking paper.
2. In a bowl, mix the almond flour, baking soda, and salt.
3. In another bowl, mix the melted coconut oil, honey or maple syrup, egg, and vanilla extract.
4. Combine the wet ingredients with the dry ingredients and mix until smooth.
5. Form balls of dough with your hands and lay them on the baking sheet, slightly flattened.
6. If you wish, you can place a whole almond in the center of each cookie.
7. Bake in the oven for about 10-12 minutes or until the cookies are golden brown.
8. Let cool before enjoying the delicious almond flour cookies.

103. Strawberry Banana Ice Cream

Ingredients for 2 persons:

- o 2 ripe frozen bananas
- o 1 cup of fresh strawberries
- o 1/4 cup coconut milk (no added sugar) or other vegetable milk

- o 1 teaspoon honey or maple syrup (optional)

Instructions:

1. Cut the frozen bananas into pieces and place them in a high-power blender.
2. Add fresh strawberries and coconut milk.
3. Blend until smooth and creamy.
4. If you want a sweet touch, you can add a teaspoon of honey or maple syrup and blend again.
5. Pour the strawberry and banana ice cream into two bowls and enjoy immediately.

104. Fruit and Yogurt Parfait.

Ingredients for 2 persons:

- o 1 cup of Greek yogurt (no added sugar) or coconut yogurt
- o 1 cup of fresh sliced strawberries
- o 1 cup of fresh blueberries
- o 1/4 cup of granola (no added sugar)
- o 1 tablespoon honey or maple syrup (optional)

Instructions:

1. In two glasses, create a layer of Greek yogurt or coconut yogurt on the bottom.
2. Add a layer of fresh sliced strawberries on top of the yogurt.
3. Continue with a layer of fresh blueberries.
4. Sprinkle granola on top of the fruit.
5. If you want a sweet touch, you can add a spoonful of honey or maple syrup on top of the granola.
6. Repeat the layers until you run out of ingredients.
7. Serve the fruit and yogurt parfaits as a light and tasty dessert.

105. Almond and Coconut Bars

Ingredients for 2 persons:

- 1 cup chopped almonds
- 1/2 cup unsweetened grated coconut
- 1/4 cup almond butter (or peanut butter)
- 1/4 cup honey or maple syrup
- 1 teaspoon vanilla extract

Instructions:

1. In a bowl, mix chopped almonds and grated coconut.
2. In a small saucepan, melt the almond butter and honey or maple syrup over medium heat, stirring until smooth.
3. Add the vanilla extract to the almond butter mixture and mix well.
4. Pour the liquid mixture over the almond and coconut mixture and stir until smooth.
5. Spread the dough on a baking sheet lined with baking paper and compact it with your hands.
6. Refrigerate for about 1 to 2 hours or until the dough becomes firm.
7. Cut the hardened dough into bars and enjoy them as a nutritious snack or dessert.

106. Coconut Flour and Lemon Cookies.

Ingredients for 2 persons:

- 1 cup of coconut flour
- 1/4 teaspoon baking soda
- 1/4 teaspoon salt
- 1 egg
- 1/4 cup honey or maple syrup
- Grated zest of 1 lemon
- Juice of 1/2 lemon

Instructions:

1. Preheat the oven to 180°C (350°F) and line a baking sheet with baking paper.

2. In a bowl, mix the coconut flour, baking soda and salt.
3. In another bowl, mix the egg, honey or maple syrup, grated zest, and lemon juice.
4. Combine the wet ingredients with the dry ingredients and mix until smooth.
5. Form balls of dough with your hands and lay them on the baking sheet, slightly flattened.
6. Bake in the oven for about 10-12 minutes or until the cookies are golden brown.
7. Let cool before enjoying the delicious coconut flour and lemon cookies.

107. Fruit and Yogurt Trifle.

Ingredients for 2 persons:

- 1 cup of Greek yogurt (no added sugar) or coconut yogurt
- 1 cup of fresh sliced strawberries
- 1 cup of fresh blueberries
- 1/2 cup granola (no added sugar)
- 1 teaspoon honey or maple syrup (optional)

Instructions:

1. In two glasses, create a layer of Greek yogurt or coconut yogurt on the bottom.
2. Add a layer of fresh sliced strawberries on top of the yogurt.
3. Continue with a layer of fresh blueberries.
4. Sprinkle the granola on top of the fruit.
5. If you want a sweet touch, you can add a teaspoon of honey or maple syrup on top of the granola.
6. Repeat the layers until you run out of ingredients.
7. Serve the fruit and yogurt trifle as a refreshing and tasty dessert.

108. Healthy Banana Split

Ingredients for 2 persons:

- 2 ripe bananas
- 1 cup of Greek yogurt (no added sugar) or coconut yogurt
- 1/4 cup of granola (no added sugar)
- 2 tablespoons maple syrup or honey
- 1/4 cup chopped walnuts
- Fresh sliced strawberries for garnish

Instructions:

1. Cut the bananas in half lengthwise and place them on a plate.
2. Spread Greek yogurt or coconut yogurt over the bananas.
3. Sprinkle the granola on top of the yogurt.
4. Add fresh strawberries on top of the granola.
5. Sprinkle chopped walnuts over the strawberries.
6. Pour maple syrup or honey over the dessert.
7. Serve the healthy banana split as a delicious and nutritious dessert.

109. Blueberry and Yogurt Ice Cream

Ingredients for 2 persons:

- 2 cups of fresh or frozen blueberries
- 1 cup of Greek yogurt (no added sugar) or coconut yogurt
- 1 teaspoon honey or maple syrup (optional)

Instructions:

1. Place the blueberries and yogurt in a high-powered blender.
2. Blend until smooth and creamy.
3. If you want a sweet touch, you can add a teaspoon of honey or maple syrup and blend again.

4. Pour the blueberry-yogurt ice cream into two bowls and enjoy immediately.

110. Coconut and Mango Mousse

Ingredients for 2 persons:

- 1 cup of coconut milk (no added sugar) or other vegetable milk
- 1 cup diced fresh mango
- 1 tablespoon honey or maple syrup (optional)
- 1 teaspoon grated coconut for garnish (optional)

Instructions:

1. In a high-power blender, blend the coconut milk and diced mango until smooth and creamy.
2. If you want a sweet touch, you can add a tablespoon of honey or maple syrup and blend again.
3. Pour the coconut-mango mousse into two bowls.
4. Garnish with grated coconut, if desired.
5. Serve the coconut and mango mousse as an exotic and light dessert.

111. Oatmeal and Coconut Cookies

Ingredients for 2 persons:

- 1 cup of oatmeal
- 1/4 cup of coconut flour
- 1/4 teaspoon baking soda
- 1/4 teaspoon salt
- 1/4 cup coconut oil (melted)
- 1/4 cup honey or maple syrup
- 1 teaspoon vanilla extract
- 1/4 cup chopped walnuts (optional)

Instructions:

1. Preheat the oven to 180°C (350°F) and line a baking sheet with baking paper.

2. In a bowl, mix oatmeal, coconut flour, baking soda and salt.
3. In another bowl, mix the melted coconut oil, honey or maple syrup, and vanilla extract.
4. Combine the wet ingredients with the dry ingredients and mix until smooth.
5. If desired, you can add chopped walnuts and mix gently.
6. Form balls of dough with your hands and lay them on the baking sheet, slightly flattened.
7. Bake in the oven for about 10-12 minutes or until the cookies are golden brown.
8. Let cool before enjoying the delicious oatmeal and coconut cookies.

Regenerating Smoothies

112. Lavender and Honey Zen Smoothie

Ingredients for 2 persons:

- 1 cup of almond milk (no added sugar) or coconut milk
- 1/2 teaspoon dried lavender
- 1 tablespoon honey (or maple syrup for vegan version)
- 1 ripe banana
- 1/2 cup fresh or frozen strawberries

Instructions:

1. Heat almond or coconut milk slightly in a saucepan over low heat.
2. Add the dried lavender to the warm milk and let it steep for a few minutes.
3. Strain the milk through a strainer to remove the lavender.
4. Place the flavored milk, honey (or maple syrup), banana and strawberries in the blender.
5. Blend until smooth and velvety.
6. Pour the lavender and honey zen smoothie into two glasses.

7. Enjoy this relaxing and rejuvenating smoothie.

113. Exotic Papaya and Lime Smoothie.

Ingredients for 2 persons:

- 1 cup fresh papaya pieces
- Juice of 1 lime
- 1/2 cup coconut milk (no added sugar) or coconut yogurt
- 1 tablespoon honey or maple syrup (optional)

Instructions:

1. Place the papaya, lime juice and coconut milk in the blender.
2. If you want a sweet touch, you can add a tablespoon of honey or maple syrup and blend again.
3. Blend until smooth and creamy.
4. Pour the exotic papaya-lime smoothie into two glasses.
5. Enjoy this delicious and rejuvenating smoothie.

114. Melon and Lime Smoothie

Ingredients for 2 persons:

- 1 cup of fresh chopped melon (cantaloupe, yellow melon or winter melon)
- Juice of 1 lime
- 1/2 cup coconut water (no added sugar) or water

Instructions:

1. Place the melon and lime juice in a blender.
2. Add coconut water or water.
3. Blend until smooth and homogeneous.
4. Pour the melon and lime smoothie into two glasses.

5. Enjoy this refreshing and rejuvenating smoothie.

115. Banana and Cocoa Smoothie

Ingredients for 2 persons:

- 2 ripe bananas
- 2 tablespoons unsweetened cocoa powder
- 1 cup of almond milk (no added sugar) or other vegetable milk
- 1 tablespoon almond butter (or other nut cream)
- Ice (optional)

Instructions:

1. Place the bananas, cocoa powder, almond milk and almond butter in the blender.
2. Blend until smooth and creamy.
3. Add ice, if desired, for a cooler drink.
4. Pour the banana and cocoa smoothie into two glasses.
5. Enjoy this delicious and rejuvenating smoothie.

116. Tropical Pineapple and Mango Smoothie.

Ingredients for 2 persons:

- 1 cup of chopped fresh pineapple
- 1 cup fresh mango pieces
- 1/2 cup coconut milk (no added sugar) or coconut yogurt
- 1/2 cup coconut water (no added sugar) or water
- 1 teaspoon of lime juice

Instructions:

1. Place the pineapple, mango, coconut milk, coconut water and lime juice in the blender.
2. Blend until smooth and homogeneous.

3. Pour the tropical pineapple-mango smoothie into two glasses.
4. Enjoy this refreshing and rejuvenating smoothie.

117. Coffee Banana Smoothie

Ingredients for 2 persons:

- 1 cup of iced coffee
- 2 ripe bananas
- 1/2 cup almond milk (no added sugar) or other vegetable milk
- 1 tablespoon almond butter (or other nut cream)
- Ice (optional)

Instructions:

1. Place the iced coffee, bananas, almond milk, and almond butter in the blender.
2. Blend until smooth and creamy.
3. Add ice, if desired, for a cooler drink.
4. Pour the coffee-banana smoothie into two glasses.
5. Enjoy this delicious and rejuvenating smoothie.

118. Energizing Smoothie with Mint and Ginger.

Ingredients for 2 persons:

- 1 cup of fresh spinach
- 1 cup of chopped fresh pineapple
- 1/2 cup fresh or frozen blueberries
- 1/2 cup coconut milk (no added sugar) or other vegetable milk
- 1 tablespoon fresh grated ginger
- Fresh mint leaves for garnish (optional)

Instructions:

1. Place the spinach, pineapple, blueberries, coconut milk and ginger in the blender.
2. Blend until smooth and creamy.

3. Pour the energizing ginger mint smoothie into two glasses.
4. Garnish with fresh mint leaves, if desired.
5. Enjoy this refreshing and rejuvenating smoothie.

119. Raspberry Vanilla Smoothie

Ingredients for 2 persons:

- o 1 cup of fresh or frozen raspberries
- o 1 cup of fresh or frozen strawberries
- o 1/2 cup Greek yogurt (no added sugar) or coconut yogurt
- o 1/2 teaspoon vanilla extract
- o Ice (optional)

Instructions:

1. Place the raspberries, strawberries, yogurt and vanilla extract in the blender.
2. Blend until smooth and creamy.
3. Add ice, if desired, for a cooler drink.
4. Pour the raspberry-vanilla smoothie into two glasses.
5. Enjoy this delicious and rejuvenating smoothie.

120. Energizing Orange and Carrot Smoothie

Ingredients for 2 persons:

- o 2 peeled and seedless oranges
- o 2 carrots peeled and cut into pieces
- o 1/2 cup coconut milk (no added sugar) or other vegetable milk
- o 1/2 teaspoon turmeric powder
- o 1/2 teaspoon cinnamon powder
- o Ice (optional)

Instructions:

1. Place the oranges, carrots, and coconut milk in the blender.
2. Add turmeric and cinnamon.

3. Blend until smooth and creamy.
4. Add ice, if desired, for a cool touch.
5. Pour the orange and carrot energizing smoothie into two glasses.
6. Enjoy this refreshing and rejuvenating smoothie.

121. Kiwi and Spinach Energizing Smoothie.

Ingredients for 2 persons:

- o 2 kiwis peeled and cut into pieces
- o 1 cup of fresh spinach
- o 1/2 cup chopped fresh pineapple
- o 1/2 cup coconut water (no added sugar) or water

Instructions:

1. Place the kiwi, spinach, pineapple and coconut water in the blender.
2. Blend until smooth and creamy.
3. Pour the energizing kiwi and spinach smoothie into two glasses.
4. Enjoy this refreshing and rejuvenating smoothie.

122. Refreshing Cherry Lemon Smoothie

Ingredients for 2 persons:

- o 1 cup of fresh or frozen cherries
- o Juice of 1 lemon
- o 1/2 cup coconut milk (no added sugar) or coconut yogurt
- o 1 teaspoon honey or maple syrup (optional)

Instructions:

1. Place the cherries and lemon juice in a blender.
2. Add the coconut milk and whisk until smooth and homogeneous.

3. If you want a sweet touch, you can add a teaspoon of honey or maple syrup and blend again.
4. Pour the refreshing cherry-lemon smoothie into two glasses.
5. Enjoy this delicious and rejuvenating smoothie.

123. Matcha and Banana Energizing Smoothie.

Ingredients for 2 persons:

- o 1 teaspoon matcha powder
- o 2 ripe bananas
- o 1 cup of almond milk (no added sugar) or other vegetable milk
- o 1 tablespoon almond butter (or other nut cream)
- o Ice (optional)

Instructions:

1. Place the matcha powder, bananas, almond milk, and almond butter in the blender.
2. Blend until smooth and creamy.
3. Add ice, if desired, for a cooler drink.
4. Pour the energizing matcha and banana smoothie into two glasses.
5. Enjoy this delicious and rejuvenating smoothie.

124. Mango Coconut Smoothie

Ingredients for 2 persons:

- o 1 cup fresh mango pieces
- o 1/2 cup coconut milk (no added sugar) or coconut yogurt
- o 1/2 cup coconut water (no added sugar) or water
- o 1/2 teaspoon vanilla extract
- o Ice (optional)

Instructions:

1. Place the mango, coconut milk, coconut water and vanilla extract in the blender.
2. Blend until smooth and creamy.
3. Add ice, if desired, for a cooler drink.
4. Pour the mango-coconut smoothie into two glasses.
5. Enjoy this refreshing and rejuvenating smoothie.

125. Celery and Cucumber Detox Smoothie

Ingredients for 2 persons:

- o 1 cup fresh chopped celery
- o 1 cup of fresh chopped cucumbers
- o 1 green apple in pieces
- o 1 cup of coconut water (no added sugar) or water

Instructions:

1. Place the celery, cucumbers, green apple and coconut water in the blender.
2. Blend until smooth and homogeneous.
3. Pour the celery and cucumber detox smoothie into two glasses.
4. Enjoy this refreshing and rejuvenating smoothie.

126. Pomegranate and Orange Invigorating Smoothie.

Ingredients for 2 persons:

- o Seeds of 1 pomegranate
- o Juice of 2 oranges
- o 1/2 cup Greek yogurt (no added sugar) or coconut yogurt
- o 1/2 teaspoon cinnamon powder

1. Place pomegranate seeds, orange juice, Greek yogurt and cinnamon in a blender.
2. Blend until smooth and creamy.
3. Pour the invigorating pomegranate-orange smoothie into two glasses.
4. Enjoy this delicious and rejuvenating smoothie.

127. Coffee and Cocoa Energy Smoothie

Ingredients for 2 persons:

- o 1 cup of iced coffee (prepared in advance and chilled)
- o 1 ripe banana
- o 2 tablespoons unsweetened cocoa powder
- o 1/2 cup almond milk (no added sugar) or other vegetable milk
- o Ice (optional)

Instructions:

1. Place the iced coffee, banana, cocoa powder and almond milk in the blender.
2. Blend until smooth and creamy.
3. Add ice, if desired, for a cooler drink.
4. Pour the coffee and cocoa energy smoothie into two glasses.
5. Enjoy this delicious and rejuvenating smoothie.

128. Refreshing Mint and Lime Smoothie.

Ingredients for 2 persons:

- o 1 cup of chopped fresh pineapple
- o Juice of 2 limes
- o Fresh mint leaves (some for the smoothie and some for garnish)
- o 1/2 cup coconut water (no added sugar) or water
- o Ice (optional)

Instructions:

1. Place the pineapple, lime juice, some mint leaves and coconut water in the blender.
2. Blend until smooth and homogeneous.
3. Add ice, if desired, for a cool touch.
4. Pour the refreshing mint and lime smoothie into two glasses.
5. Garnish with fresh mint leaves, if desired.
6. Enjoy this refreshing and rejuvenating smoothie.

129. Green Tea Ginger Energy Smoothie.

Ingredients for 2 persons:

- o 1 cup of iced green tea (prepared in advance and chilled)
- o 1 ripe banana
- o 1 tablespoon fresh grated ginger
- o 1/2 cup coconut milk (no added sugar) or other vegetable milk
- o Honey or maple syrup for sweetening, if desired (optional)
- o Ice (optional)

Instructions:

1. Place the iced green tea, banana, ginger and coconut milk in the blender.
2. If you want a sweet touch, you can add a little honey or maple syrup and blend again.
3. Add ice, if desired, for a cooler drink.
4. Pour the green tea and ginger energy smoothie into two glasses.
5. Enjoy this delicious and rejuvenating smoothie.

130. Goji Berry and Blueberry Antioxidant Smoothie.

Ingredients for 2 persons:

- o 1 cup of fresh or frozen blueberries

- 1/4 cup dried goji berries (soaked in hot water for 10 minutes and then drained)
- 1/2 cup almond milk (no added sugar) or other vegetable milk
- 1 tablespoon of chia seeds
- Ice (optional)

Instructions:

1. Place the blueberries, goji berries, almond milk and chia seeds in the blender.
2. Blend until smooth and creamy.
3. Add ice, if desired, for a cooler drink.
4. Pour the antioxidant goji berry and blueberry smoothie into two glasses.
5. Enjoy this refreshing and rejuvenating smoothie.

131. Turmeric Chicken Meatballs.

Ingredients for 2 servings:

- ounces of ground chicken breast
- 1 teaspoon turmeric powder
- 1/4 teaspoon salt
- 1/4 teaspoon black pepper
- 1 tablespoon of olive oil

Instructions:

1. In a bowl, mix ground chicken breast with turmeric, salt, and black pepper.
2. Form small patties with your hands.
3. Heat the olive oil in a nonstick skillet and cook the meatballs until well cooked and golden brown on both sides.
4. Serve turmeric chicken meatballs as a main dish or snack.

132. Whole Grain Pasta with Tomato and Basil Sauce.

Ingredients for 2 servings:

- oncedi whole wheat pasta (choice of penne, fusilli or farfalle)

- 1 cup of tomato sauce (no added sugar)
- Fresh basil leaves
- Salt and pepper to taste.

Instructions:

1. Cook whole wheat pasta in plenty of salted water following the instructions on the package.
2. Heat the tomato sauce in a frying pan.
3. Drain the cooked al dente pasta and add it to the tomato sauce, mixing well.
4. Add fresh basil leaves and season with salt and pepper to taste.
5. Serve whole wheat pasta with tomato basil sauce.

133. Grilled Chicken with Sweet Potatoes.

Ingredients for 2 servings:

- 2 chicken breasts
- 2 medium sweet potatoes, peeled and thinly sliced
- 1 tablespoon of olive oil
- Salt and pepper to taste.

Instructions:

1. Preheat a grill and brush the chicken breasts with olive oil.
2. Grill the chicken breasts until cooked through, turning them occasionally.
3. Meanwhile, blanch sweet potato slices on a grill or in a nonstick skillet until tender and slightly crisp.
4. Season the chicken and sweet potatoes with salt and pepper to taste.
5. Serve grilled chicken with sweet potatoes as a main dish.

134. Mini Wholewheat Pizzas

Ingredients for 2 servings:

- o 2 whole wheat pizza bases (or whole wheat pita)
- o 1/2 cup tomato sauce (no added sugar)
- o 1/2 cup of grated mozzarella cheese (lactose-free, if needed)
- o Vegetables of your choice (such as sliced tomatoes, peppers, mushrooms, zucchini)
- o Fresh basil leaves
- o Salt and pepper to taste.

Instructions:

1. Preheat the oven to 200°C (390°F).
2. Arrange the whole-wheat pizza bases on a baking sheet lined with baking paper.
3. Spread the tomato sauce on the surface of the pizza bases.
4. Add grated mozzarella cheese and vegetables of your choice.
5. Season with salt and pepper to taste.
6. Bake the mini pizzas for about 10 to 15 minutes or until the cheese is melted and lightly browned.
7. Serve the mini whole-wheat pizzas with fresh basil leaves.

135. Hummus with Carrots and Celery

Ingredients for 2 servings:

- o 1 cup of cooked chickpeas (rinsed and drained)
- o 2 tablespoons of tahina (sesame seed paste)
- o Juice of 1/2 lemon
- o 1 clove of garlic
- o 2 tablespoons of olive oil
- o Salt and pepper to taste.
- o Carrots and celery for serving

Instructions:

1. Place the cooked chickpeas, tahina, lemon juice, garlic clove, olive oil, salt, and pepper in a blender.
2. Blend until smooth and creamy.
3. Transfer hummus to a bowl and serve with carrots and celery cut into sticks.

136. Quinoa with Broccoli and Walnuts.

Ingredients for 2 servings:

- o 1 cup of cooked quinoa
- o 1 cup steamed or boiled broccoli
- o 1/4 cup chopped walnuts
- o 1 tablespoon of olive oil
- o Salt and pepper to taste.

Instructions:

1. Heat olive oil in a skillet and add steamed or boiled broccoli.
2. Saute broccoli for a few minutes until well seasoned with oil.
3. Add the cooked quinoa to the pan with the broccoli and mix well.
4. Season with salt and pepper to taste.
5. Add chopped walnuts and stir again.
6. Serve quinoa with broccoli and walnuts as a side or main dish.

137. Herb Omelette with Spinach

Ingredients for 2 servings:

- o 4 eggs
- o 1 cup of fresh spinach
- o 2 tablespoons chopped herbs (parsley, basil, chives)
- o 1/4 teaspoon turmeric powder
- o Salt and pepper to taste.
- o Olive oil to taste.

Instructions:

1. In a bowl, beat the eggs with the chopped herbs, turmeric, salt and pepper.
2. Heat some olive oil in a nonstick frying pan.
3. Pour the egg mixture into the hot pan.
4. Add fresh spinach on top of the eggs.
5. Cook over medium-low heat until the eggs are well cooked and the omelet has turned a golden color.
6. Cut the herb omelet with spinach into slices and serve as a main dish or snack.

138. Whole grain sandwiches with Chicken and Avocado

Ingredients for 2 servings:

- 2 whole-grain sandwiches
- ounces of grilled or baked chicken breast
- 1 ripe avocado, sliced
- Fresh lettuce leaves
- Sliced tomatoes
- Mustard (no added sugar) or light mayonnaise (optional)

Instructions:

1. Cut the whole wheat rolls in half and open them.
2. Fill the sandwiches with grilled or baked chicken breast.
3. Add avocado slices, lettuce leaves, and tomato slices.
4. Spread mustard or light mayonnaise on the sandwiches, if desired.
5. Close the sandwiches and serve them as lunch or light dinner.

139. Vegetable Minestrone

Ingredients for 2 servings:

- 1 carrot, diced

- 1 celery, diced
- 1 potato, diced
- 1 zucchini, diced
- 1/2 onion, chopped
- 2 cloves of garlic, minced
- 1 l vegetable broth (without MSG)
- 1 cup chopped peeled tomatoes (canned, no added sugar)
- 1 cup cooked cannellini beans (canned, rinsed and drained)
- 1 tablespoon of olive oil
- 1 tablespoon fresh chopped parsley
- Salt and pepper to taste.

Instructions:

1. Heat olive oil in a pot and add chopped onion and garlic. Sauté until they are lightly browned.
2. Add the diced carrots, celery, potatoes, and zucchini to the pot. Brown the vegetables for a few minutes.
3. Pour the vegetable broth into the pot and bring to a boil.
4. Reduce the flame and simmer for about 15-20 minutes, or until the vegetables are tender.
5. Add the peeled tomatoes and cooked cannellini beans. Continue to cook for another 5 minutes.
6. Season with salt and pepper to taste.
7. Before serving, sprinkle the vegetable soup with chopped fresh parsley.

140. Steamed Broccoli with Lemon Yogurt Sauce.

Ingredients for 2 servings:

- 2 cups fresh broccoli, cut into florets
- 1/2 cup Greek yogurt (no added sugar)
- Juice and zest of 1/2 lemon
- 1 clove of garlic, minced
- Salt and pepper to taste.

Instructions:

1. In a steamer pot, cook fresh broccoli until tender but crisp.
2. In a bowl, mix Greek yogurt with lemon juice and zest, minced garlic, salt and pepper.
3. Season the steamed broccoli with the lemon yogurt sauce before serving.

141. Turkey and Avocado Wrap

Ingredients for 2 servings:

- o 2 whole wheat or corn tortillas
- o 7 ounces of sliced turkey
- o 1 ripe avocado, sliced
- o Fresh spinach leaves
- o 1/2 cucumber, thinly sliced
- o 1 tablespoon light mayonnaise (no added sugar, optional)

Instructions:

1. Heat whole wheat or corn tortillas in a nonstick skillet until hot and pliable.
2. Arrange the turkey slices in the center of each tortilla.
3. Add the avocado slices, spinach leaves, and cucumber slices.
4. Spread light mayonnaise on the tortillas, if desired.
5. Roll the tortillas tightly, folding the sides inward to close the wraps.
6. Cut each wrap in half and serve as a light lunch or dinner.

142. Chickpea and Tomato Salad

Ingredients for 2 servings:

- o 1 can of cooked chickpeas (rinsed and drained)
- o 1 cup cherry tomatoes, cut in half
- o 1 cucumber, diced

- o 1/4 red onion, thinly sliced
- o Fresh basil leaves
- o 1 tablespoon of olive oil
- o Juice of 1/2 lemon
- o Salt and pepper to taste.

Instructions:

1. In a bowl, mix the cooked chickpeas with the cherry tomatoes, cucumber, red onion, and fresh basil leaves.
2. Season with olive oil, lemon juice, salt and pepper to taste.
3. Mix all ingredients well.
4. Serve the chickpea and tomato salad as a side dish or main course.

143. Brown Rice with Bell Peppers and Zucchini

Ingredients for 2 servings:

- o 1 cup of cooked brown rice
- o 1 red bell pepper, diced
- o 1 zucchini, diced
- o 1/2 onion, chopped
- o 2 tablespoons of olive oil
- o Salt and pepper to taste.

Instructions:

1. Heat olive oil in a frying pan and add chopped onion.
2. Brown the onion until golden brown.
3. Add the diced peppers and zucchini to the pan with the onion and saute the vegetables until tender.
4. Add the cooked brown rice to the pan with the sautéed vegetables and stir well.
5. Season with salt and pepper to taste.
6. Serve brown rice with peppers and zucchini as a main dish or side dish.

144. Baked Vegetarian Meatballs

Ingredients for 2 servings:

- 1 cup of cooked chickpeas (rinsed and drained)
- 1/2 cup oatmeal or almond meal
- 1/4 cup grated carrots
- 1/4 cup grated zucchini
- 1 clove of garlic, minced
- 1 tablespoon of olive oil
- 1 tablespoon fresh chopped parsley
- 1/2 teaspoon cumin powder
- 1/2 teaspoon sweet paprika
- Salt and pepper to taste.

Instructions:

1. Preheat the oven to 200°C (390°F) and line a baking sheet with baking paper.
2. In a food processor, chop the cooked chickpeas to a coarse consistency.
3. Transfer chopped chickpeas to a bowl and add oatmeal or almond flour, grated carrots, grated zucchini, minced garlic clove, olive oil, chopped fresh parsley, cumin powder, sweet paprika, salt, and pepper.
4. Mix all ingredients well until smooth.
5. Form small patties with your hands and place them on the baking sheet lined with baking paper.
6. Bake the meatballs for about 20-25 minutes or until golden brown and crispy.
7. Serve baked vegetarian meatballs as a main dish or snack.

145. Fresh Fruit Salad

Ingredients for 2 servings:

- 1 apple, diced
- 1 pear, diced
- 1 cup fresh strawberries, cut into pieces
- 1/2 cup grapes, cut in half
- Juice of 1/2 lemon
- Fresh mint leaves

Instructions:

1. In a bowl, mix the chopped apple, pear, strawberries and grapes.
2. Season the fruit with lemon juice and mix well.
3. Add a few fresh mint leaves on top of the fruit before serving.
4. Serve the fresh fruit salad as a dessert or healthy snack.

146. Whole Grain Pasta with Dried Tomatoes and Spinach

Ingredients for 2 servings:

- ounces of whole wheat pasta (choice of penne, fusilli or farfalle)
- 1/4 cup dried tomatoes in oil, chopped
- 2 handfuls of fresh spinach leaves
- 1 tablespoon of olive oil
- 1 clove of garlic, minced
- Salt and pepper to taste.

Instructions:

1. Cook whole wheat pasta in plenty of salted water following the instructions on the package.
2. Heat olive oil in a frying pan and add the minced garlic clove.
3. Brown the garlic until golden brown.
4. Add chopped sun-dried tomatoes and fresh spinach leaves to the pan with browned garlic.
5. Saute the ingredients until the spinach has wilted and the sun-dried tomatoes are well seasoned with oil.
6. Drain the cooked al dente pasta and add it to the pan with the sautéed ingredients.
7. Mix all ingredients well and season with salt and pepper to taste.
8. Serve whole wheat pasta with sun-dried tomatoes and spinach as a main dish.

147. Basmati Rice Salad with Almonds and Raisins.

Ingredients for 2 servings:

- o 1 cup of cooked basmati rice
- o 1/4 cup toasted almonds, chopped
- o 1/4 cup of raisins
- o 1 tablespoon of olive oil
- o Juice of 1/2 lemon
- o 1 teaspoon of honey (optional)
- o Salt and pepper to taste.

Instructions:

1. In a bowl, mix cooked basmati rice with chopped toasted almonds and raisins.
2. In a small bowl, mix the olive oil, lemon juice and honey (if using) to make the vinaigrette.
3. Dress the rice salad with the vinaigrette and mix all the ingredients well.
4. Season with salt and pepper to taste.
5. Serve basmati rice salad with almonds and raisins as a side or main dish.

148. Red Lentil Soup with Carrots and Celery.

Ingredients for 2 servings:

- o 1 cup dried red lentils
- o 1 carrot, diced
- o 1 celery stalk, diced
- o 1/2 onion, chopped
- o 2 cloves of garlic, minced
- o 1 liter of vegetable broth (without MSG)
- o 1 tablespoon of olive oil
- o 1 teaspoon turmeric powder
- o 1/2 teaspoon cumin powder
- o Salt and pepper to taste.

Instructions:

1. Heat olive oil in a pot and add chopped onion and garlic. Sauté until they are lightly browned.
2. Add the diced carrots and celery to the pot with the onion and garlic and saute the vegetables until tender.
3. Add the dried red lentils to the pot with the sautéed vegetables and stir well.
4. Pour the vegetable broth into the pot and bring to a boil.
5. Reduce the heat and simmer for about 15-20 minutes or until the lentils are cooked and tender.
6. Add turmeric powder and cumin powder to season the soup.
7. Season with salt and pepper to taste.
8. Serve red lentil soup with carrots and celery as a main dish or as a side dish.

149. Avocado and Tomato Toast.

Ingredients for 2 servings:

- o 2 slices of whole wheat bread
- o 1 ripe avocado, crushed
- o 1 ripe tomato, sliced
- o Fresh basil leaves
- o 1 tablespoon of olive oil
- o Salt and pepper to taste.

Instructions:

1. Toast the slices of whole-wheat bread.
2. Spread the mashed avocado on the toasted bread slices.
3. Arrange tomato slices and fresh basil leaves on bread slices with avocado.
4. Season with olive oil, salt and pepper to taste.
5. Serve avocado and tomato toast as a snack or savory breakfast.

150. Pumpkin Hummus

Ingredients for 2 servings:

- o 1 cup cooked and mashed pumpkin
- o 1 cup of cooked chickpeas (rinsed and drained)
- o 2 tablespoons of tahina (sesame seed paste)
- o Juice of 1/2 lemon
- o 1 clove of garlic
- o 2 tablespoons of olive oil
- o Sweet paprika (for garnish)
- o Salt and pepper to taste.

Instructions:

1. Place cooked and mashed pumpkin, cooked chickpeas, tahina, lemon juice, garlic clove, and olive oil in blender.
2. Blend until smooth and creamy.
3. Transfer the pumpkin hummus to a bowl and season with salt and pepper to taste.
4. Sprinkle with sweet paprika for garnish.
5. Serve pumpkin hummus with carrot and celery sticks or with whole wheat bread as a snack or appetizer.

151. Spinach Salad with Strawberries and Almonds.

Ingredients for 2 servings:

- o 2 handfuls of fresh spinach leaves
- o 1 cup fresh strawberries, cut into slices
- o 2 tablespoons chopped toasted almonds
- o 1 tablespoon of olive oil
- o 1 tablespoon balsamic vinegar
- o 1 teaspoon of honey (optional)
- o Salt and pepper to taste.

Instructions:

1. In a bowl, mix fresh spinach leaves with sliced strawberries.

2. Add chopped toasted almonds to the surface of the salad.
3. In a small container, mix the olive oil, balsamic vinegar and honey (if using) to make the vinaigrette.
4. Dress the spinach salad with strawberries and almonds with the vinaigrette and mix all the ingredients well.
5. Season with salt and pepper to taste.
6. Serve spinach salad with strawberries and almonds as a side dish or main course.

152. Baked Salmon with Vegetables

Ingredients for 2 servings:

- o 2 salmon fillets
- o 1 zucchini, thinly sliced
- o 1 carrot, thinly sliced
- o 1 lemon, sliced
- o 2 tablespoons of olive oil
- o Salt and pepper to taste.

Instructions:

1. Preheat the oven to 200°C (390°F) and line a baking sheet with baking paper.
2. Place the salmon fillets on the baking sheet.
3. Arrange the zucchini and carrot slices on the salmon fillets.
4. Lay the lemon slices on top of the vegetables and salmon.
5. Season with olive oil, salt and pepper to taste.
6. Bake for about 15 to 20 minutes or until the salmon is well cooked and the vegetables are tender.
7. Serve the baked salmon with vegetables as a main dish.

153. Potato Salad with Smoked Salmon

Ingredients for 2 servings:

- o 2 medium red potatoes, boiled and diced

- o ounces of smoked salmon, cut into strips
- o 1/4 red onion, thinly sliced
- o Capers (optional)
- o Chopped fresh parsley
- o 1 tablespoon of olive oil
- o Juice of 1/2 lemon
- o Salt and pepper to taste.

Instructions:

1. In a bowl, mix the boiled and diced red potatoes with the smoked salmon cut into strips.
2. Add the thinly sliced red onion and capers, if used.
3. Dress the potato salad with smoked salmon with olive oil and lemon juice.
4. Mix all ingredients well.
5. Sprinkle with chopped fresh parsley for garnish.
6. Serve potato salad with smoked salmon as a main dish or side dish.

154. Guacamole sauce

Ingredients for 2 servings:

- o 1 ripe avocado
- o 1/2 ripe tomato, diced
- o 1/4 red onion, finely chopped
- o Juice of 1/2 lemon
- o 1 clove of garlic, minced
- o Chopped red chili pepper (optional)
- o Salt and pepper to taste.

Instructions:

1. In a bowl, mash the ripe avocado with a fork until creamy.
2. Add diced tomato, finely chopped red onion, chopped garlic clove and chopped red chili pepper, if used.
3. Season the guacamole sauce with lemon juice, salt and pepper to taste.
4. Mix all ingredients well.

5. Serve guacamole salsa with whole-grain nachos or as a side dish for meat or fish dishes.

155. Tofu with Sautéed Vegetables

Ingredients for 2 servings:

- o 1 cup tofu, cut into cubes
- o 1 zucchini, thinly sliced
- o 1 red bell pepper, cut into strips
- o 1/4 red onion, thinly sliced
- o 2 tablespoons soy sauce (MSG-free)
- o 1 tablespoon of olive oil
- o Salt and pepper to taste.

Instructions:

1. Heat olive oil in a frying pan and add the thinly sliced red onion.
2. Brown the onion until golden brown.
3. Add the zucchini slices and bell bell pepper strips to the pan with the onion and saute the vegetables until tender.
4. Add the tofu cubes to the pan with the sautéed vegetables and stir well.
5. Season with soy sauce, salt and pepper to taste.
6. Serve tofu with sautéed vegetables as a main dish or side dish.

156. Watermelon and Strawberry Smoothie

Ingredients for 2 servings:

- o 2 cups seedless watermelon, cut into cubes
- o 1 cup fresh strawberries, cut into pieces
- o Juice of 1/2 lemon
- o Fresh mint leaves

Instructions:

1. In a blender, mix diced watermelon with chopped strawberries.

2. Add the lemon juice to the blender.
3. Blend until smooth and homogeneous.
4. Pour the watermelon-strawberry smoothie into glasses and garnish with fresh mint leaves.
5. Serve the smoothie as a refreshing and thirst-quenching drink.

157. Couscous with Chickpeas and Vegetables.

Ingredients for 2 servings:

- 1 cup precooked couscous
- 1 can of cooked chickpeas (rinsed and drained)
- 1 zucchini, diced
- 1 carrot, diced
- 1/4 red onion, finely chopped
- 1 clove of garlic, minced
- 1 tablespoon of olive oil
- 1 teaspoon cumin powder
- 1 teaspoon sweet paprika
- Salt and pepper to taste.

Instructions:

1. Prepare the precooked couscous according to the instructions on the package.
2. Heat olive oil in a frying pan and add finely chopped red onion and chopped garlic clove.
3. Brown the onion and garlic until golden brown.
4. Add the diced zucchini and carrot to the pan with the onion and garlic and saute the vegetables until tender.
5. Add the cooked chickpeas to the pan with the sautéed vegetables and mix well.
6. Season with cumin powder, sweet paprika, salt and pepper to taste.
7. Serve couscous with chickpeas and vegetables as a main dish or side dish.

158. Whole Grain Pancakes with Blueberries

Ingredients for 2 servings:

- 1 cup of whole wheat flour
- 1 teaspoon baking powder
- 1/2 teaspoon baking soda
- 1 tablespoon of brown sugar (optional)
- 1 cup of milk (or vegetable milk)
- 1 egg (or vegan substitute, if needed)
- 1 tablespoon of olive oil
- Fresh blueberries (or other berries) for garnish

Instructions:

1. In a bowl, mix the whole wheat flour, baking powder, baking soda, and brown sugar (if using).
2. In another bowl, beat the egg (or vegan substitute) with the milk and olive oil.
3. Pour the liquid mixture into the bowl with the dry ingredients and mix well until smooth.
4. Heat a nonstick skillet and pour in a ladleful of batter to form a pancake.
5. Add some fresh blueberries to the surface of the pancake.
6. Cook the pancake until bubbles form on the surface and the edges are golden brown. Then flip the pancake over and cook the other side until cooked through.
7. Repeat the process with the remaining dough to make the other pancakes.
8. Serve whole-wheat pancakes with blueberries with maple syrup or honey (optional) as a breakfast or snack.

159. Quinoa Salad with Cucumbers and Tomatoes.

Ingredients for 2 servings:

- 1 cup of cooked quinoa

- o 1 cucumber, diced
- o 1 cup cherry tomatoes, cut in half
- o 1/4 red onion, thinly sliced
- o Chopped fresh parsley leaves
- o 1 tablespoon of olive oil
- o Juice of 1/2 lemon
- o Salt and pepper to taste.

Instructions:

1. In a bowl, mix cooked quinoa with diced cucumber, halved cherry tomatoes, and thinly sliced red onion.
2. Add chopped fresh parsley to the surface of the quinoa salad.
3. Dress the quinoa salad with cucumbers and tomatoes with olive oil and lemon juice.
4. Mix all ingredients well.
5. Season with salt and pepper to taste.
6. Serve the quinoa salad as a main dish or side dish.

160. Chicken and Zucchini Patties.

Ingredients for 2 servings:

- o 7 ounces of chopped chicken breast
- o 1 zucchini, grated
- o 1/4 red onion, finely chopped
- o 1 clove of garlic, minced
- o 1 tablespoon breadcrumbs
- o 1 egg (or vegan substitute, if needed)
- o 1 tablespoon of olive oil
- o Salt and pepper to taste.

Instructions:

1. In a bowl, mix chopped chicken breast with grated zucchini, finely chopped red onion, and minced garlic clove.
2. Add the breadcrumbs and egg (or vegan substitute) and mix all ingredients well until smooth.
3. Form small patties with your hands.
4. Heat olive oil in a skillet and add the chicken and zucchini patties.

5. Cook the patties over medium heat until well cooked and golden brown on all sides.
6. Season with salt and pepper to taste.
7. Serve the chicken and zucchini patties as a main dish or side dish.

161. Whole Grain Tostadas with Black Beans and Guacamole.

Ingredients for 2 servings:

- o 4 whole grain tostadas (or corn tortillas)
- o 1 can of cooked black beans (rinsed and drained)
- o Guacamole (see recipe under 154)
- o 1 ripe tomato, diced
- o 1/4 red onion, finely chopped
- o Fresh coriander leaves

Instructions:

1. Heat whole grain tostadas (or corn tortillas) in a nonstick skillet until hot and crispy.
2. Spread the guacamole on each tostada.
3. Add the cooked black beans on top of the guacamole.
4. Arrange the tomato cubes and finely chopped red onion on top of the black beans.
5. Garnish with fresh coriander leaves.
6. Serve whole grain tostadas with black beans and guacamole as a light lunch or dinner.

162. Couscous Salad with Grilled Vegetables.

Ingredients for 2 servings:

- o 1 cup precooked couscous
- o 1 small zucchini, thinly sliced
- o 1 yellow bell pepper, cut into strips
- o 1 eggplant, thinly sliced

- 1/4 red onion, thinly sliced
- 2 tablespoons of olive oil
- Juice of 1 lemon
- Chopped fresh parsley
- Salt and pepper to taste.

Instructions:

1. Prepare the couscous following the instructions on the package.
2. Heat a grill or nonstick skillet over medium-high heat.
3. Brush the zucchini, bell bell pepper, and eggplant slices with olive oil and grill them until tender and lightly browned on both sides.
4. In a bowl, mix the couscous with the grilled vegetables and thinly sliced red onion.
5. Season with lemon juice, fresh chopped parsley, salt and pepper.
6. Mix all ingredients well.
7. Store couscous salad with grilled vegetables in airtight containers and take it to work for a light and nutritious lunch.

163. Turkey and Avocado Wrap.

Ingredients for 2 servings:

- 4 whole wheat tortillas
- 7 ounces of sliced turkey
- 1 ripe avocado, peeled and sliced
- Fresh lettuce
- Sliced tomatoes
- 2 tablespoons of vegan mayonnaise
- Juice of 1 lemon
- Salt and pepper to taste.

Instructions:

1. Heat whole wheat tortillas slightly on the grill or in the microwave to make them soft and pliable.
2. Spread a tablespoon of vegan mayonnaise on each tortilla.

3. Add turkey slices, avocado, fresh lettuce, and sliced tomatoes to the center of each tortilla.
4. Season with lemon juice, salt and pepper to taste.
5. Roll the tortillas tightly and wrap them in aluminum foil or plastic wrap to take to work.

164. Basmati Rice Salad with Black Beans.

Ingredients for 2 servings:

- 1 cup of cooked basmati rice
- 1 can of cooked, rinsed and drained black beans
- 1/2 cup sweet corn
- 1/4 cup mixed peppers, diced
- 1/4 cup red onion, thinly sliced
- 2 tablespoons of olive oil
- Juice of 1 lemon
- Chopped fresh coriander
- Salt and pepper to taste.

Instructions:

1. In a bowl, mix cooked basmati rice with black beans, sweet corn, mixed peppers, and thinly sliced red onion.
2. Season with olive oil and lemon juice.
3. Add chopped fresh cilantro and mix all ingredients well.
4. Season with salt and pepper to taste.
5. Store basmati rice salad with black beans in airtight containers and bring it to work for a tasty, protein-packed lunch.

165. Vegan Curry Wrap

Ingredients for 2 servings:

- 4 whole wheat tortillas
- 1 cup of cooked chickpeas, mashed with a fork

- 1/2 ripe avocado, mashed with a fork
- 1/4 cup grated carrots
- 1/4 cup red cabbage, cut into thin strips
- 2 tablespoons of vegan mayonnaise
- 1 teaspoon curry powder
- Juice of 1 lemon
- Salt and pepper to taste.

Instructions:

1. Heat whole wheat tortillas slightly on the grill or in the microwave to make them soft and pliable.
2. In a bowl, mix crushed chickpeas, mashed avocado, grated carrots, and red cabbage cut into thin strips.
3. Season with vegan mayonnaise, curry powder and lemon juice.
4. Mix all ingredients well and season with salt and pepper to taste.
5. Spread the curry mixture over each tortilla and roll tightly.
6. Wrap the vegan curry wraps in aluminum foil or plastic wrap to take to work.

166. Quinoa Salad with Fresh Vegetables.

Ingredients for 2 servings:

- 1 cup of cooked quinoa
- 1 cucumber, diced
- 1 red bell pepper, diced
- 1 tomato, diced
- 1/4 cup black olives, pitted and sliced
- 2 tablespoons of olive oil
- 1 tablespoon apple cider vinegar
- Chopped fresh parsley
- Salt and pepper to taste.

Instructions:

1. In a bowl, mix the cooked quinoa with the cucumber, red bell pepper, tomato, and sliced black olives.
2. Season with olive oil and apple cider vinegar.

3. Add fresh chopped parsley and mix all ingredients well.
4. Season with salt and pepper to taste.
5. Store quinoa salad with fresh vegetables in airtight containers and take it to work for a light, nutritious lunch.

167. Vegetarian Club Sandwich

Ingredients for 2 servings:

- 6 slices of whole wheat bread
- 4 lettuce leaves
- 1 tomato, sliced
- 1/2 ripe avocado, sliced
- 4 slices of vegan cheddar cheese
- 4 slices of smoked tofu
- 2 tablespoons of vegan mayonnaise
- 1 teaspoon of mustard
- Salt and pepper to taste.

Instructions:

1. Toast the slices of whole-wheat bread lightly.
1. Spread vegan mayonnaise on a slice of toast.
2. Overlap a lettuce leaf, a slice of smoked tofu, a slice of vegan cheddar cheese, and a few slices of avocado.
3. Spread mustard on a second slice of toast and place it on top of the previous ingredients.
4. Continue the same process to create a second layer of ingredients.
5. Cover with the last slice of toast.
6. Cut the veggie club sandwich in half and store it in plastic wrap to take to work.

168. Lentil and Avocado Salad.

Ingredients for 2 servings:

- 1 cup of cooked lentils
- 1 ripe avocado, cut into cubes
- 1/4 cup red onion, thinly sliced

- 1/4 cup cucumber, diced
- 2 tablespoons of olive oil
- Juice of 1 lemon
- Chopped fresh thyme
- Salt and pepper to taste.

Instructions:

1. In a bowl, mix cooked lentils with diced avocado, thinly sliced red onion, and diced cucumber.
2. Season with olive oil and lemon juice.
3. Add chopped fresh thyme and mix all ingredients well.
4. Season with salt and pepper to taste.
5. Store the lentil and avocado salad in airtight containers and bring it to work for a nutritious and tasty lunch.

169. Quinoa and Avocado Salad.

Ingredients for 2 servings:

- 1 cup of cooked quinoa
- 1 ripe avocado, cut into cubes
- 1/4 cup mixed peppers, diced
- 1/4 cup cucumber, diced
- 2 tablespoons of olive oil
- Juice of 1 lemon
- Chopped fresh basil
- Salt and pepper to taste.

Instructions:

1. In a bowl, mix cooked quinoa with diced avocado, diced mixed peppers, and diced cucumber.
2. Season with olive oil and lemon juice.
3. Add chopped fresh basil and mix all ingredients well.
4. Season with salt and pepper to taste.
5. Store the quinoa and avocado salad in airtight containers and bring it to work for a light and tasty lunch.

170. Vegan Wrap with Hummus and Vegetables.

Ingredients for 2 servings:

- 2 whole wheat tortillas
- 1/2 cup hummus
- 1 carrot, cut into julienne strips
- 1 cucumber, cut into julienne strips
- 1/2 ripe avocado, cut into slices
- 1/4 cup cherry tomatoes, cut in half
- Lettuce leaves

Instructions:

1. Roll out the whole wheat tortillas on a work surface.
2. Spread the hummus evenly on both tortillas.
3. Arrange julienned carrots, julienned cucumbers, avocado slices, and cherry tomatoes on the bottom half of each tortilla.
4. Add some lettuce leaves and close the wraps by rolling them tightly.
5. Cut each wrap in half and wrap them in food-grade paper to take to work.

171. Spelt and Cucumber Salad

Ingredients for 2 servings:

- 1 cup of cooked spelt
- 1 cucumber, diced
- 1/4 cup red onion, thinly sliced
- 1/4 cup black olives, pitted and sliced
- 2 tablespoons of olive oil
- 1 tablespoon apple cider vinegar
- Chopped fresh mint
- Salt and pepper to taste.

Instructions:

1. In a bowl, mix cooked farro with diced cucumber, thinly sliced red onion, and sliced black olives.

2. Season with olive oil and apple cider vinegar.
3. Add chopped fresh mint and mix all ingredients well.
4. Season with salt and pepper to taste.
5. Store the spelt and cucumber salad in airtight containers and bring it to work for a nutritious and tasty lunch.

172. Quinoa and Avocado Salad with Black Beans.

Ingredients for 2 servings:

- o 1 cup of cooked quinoa
- o 1 ripe avocado, cut into cubes
- o 1/2 cup of cooked black beans
- o 1/4 cup mixed peppers, diced
- o 2 tablespoons of olive oil
- o Juice of 1 lime
- o Chopped fresh coriander
- o Salt and pepper to taste.

Instructions:

1. In a bowl, mix cooked quinoa with diced avocado, cooked black beans, and diced mixed peppers.
2. Dress with olive oil and lime juice.
3. Add chopped fresh cilantro and mix all ingredients well.
4. Season with salt and pepper to taste.
5. Store the quinoa and avocado salad with black beans in airtight containers and bring it to work for a light and tasty lunch.

173. Lettuce Wraps with Tofu and Vegetables.

Ingredients for 2 servings:

- o Large lettuce leaves, washed and dried
- o ounces of tofu, diced
- o 1/2 cup mixed peppers, cut into thin strips

- o 1/2 cup carrots, cut into julienne strips
- o 1/4 cup red onion, thinly sliced
- o Sodium-reduced soy sauce
- o 2 tablespoons of olive oil
- o Toasted sesame (optional)

Instructions:

1. Place the lettuce leaves on a plate and spread the tofu, mixed peppers, carrots, and red onion on the bottom of each leaf.
2. Drizzle some reduced sodium soy sauce and olive oil over the vegetables.
3. Roll the lettuce leaves to create wraps and secure them with a toothpick.
4. Sprinkle with toasted sesame (optional) and store lettuce wraps with tofu and vegetables in an airtight container to take to work.

174. Barley and Chickpea Salad

Ingredients for 2 servings:

- o 1 cup of cooked barley
- o 1 cup of cooked chickpeas
- o 1/2 cup cherry tomatoes, cut in half
- o 1/4 cup black olives, pitted and sliced
- o 1/4 cup cucumber, diced
- o 2 tablespoons of olive oil
- o Juice of 1 lemon
- o Chopped fresh oregano
- o Salt and pepper to taste.

Instructions:

1. In a bowl, mix the cooked barley with the cooked chickpeas, halved cherry tomatoes, sliced black olives, and diced cucumber.
2. Season with olive oil and lemon juice.
3. Add fresh chopped oregano and mix all ingredients well.
4. Season with salt and pepper to taste.
5. Store the barley and chickpea salad in airtight containers and bring it to work for a nutritious and tasty lunch.

175. Vegan Sandwich with Hummus and Grilled Vegetables.

Ingredients for 2 servings:

- 2 whole-grain vegan sandwiches
- 1/2 cup hummus
- 1 zucchini, thinly sliced
- 1 eggplant, thinly sliced
- 1 red bell pepper, cut into strips
- 2 tablespoons of olive oil
- Salt and pepper to taste.
- Arugula

Instructions:

1. Preheat a nonstick grill or frying pan.
2. Brush the zucchini, eggplant, and bell bell pepper slices with olive oil and season with salt and pepper.
3. Grill vegetables until tender and slightly charred.
4. Cut the vegan sandwiches in half and spread hummus on both sides.
5. Fill the sandwiches with the grilled vegetables and a few arugula leaves.
6. Close the sandwiches and store them in plastic wrap to take to work.

176. Mediterranean Couscous Salad

Ingredients for 2 servings:

- 1 cup of cooked couscous
- 1/2 cup of cooked chickpeas
- 1/4 cup cherry tomatoes, cut in half
- 1/4 cup cucumber, diced
- 1/4 cup mixed peppers, diced
- 2 tablespoons of olive oil
- Juice of 1 lemon
- Chopped fresh mint
- Salt and pepper to taste.

Instructions:

1. In a bowl, mix cooked couscous with cooked chickpeas, halved cherry tomatoes, diced cucumber, and diced mixed peppers.
2. Season with olive oil and lemon juice.
3. Add chopped fresh mint and mix all ingredients well.
4. Season with salt and pepper to taste.
5. Store Mediterranean couscous salad in airtight containers and bring it to work for a light and tasty lunch.

177. Brown Rice and Avocado Salad.

Ingredients for 2 servings:

- 1 cup of cooked brown rice
- 1 ripe avocado, cut into cubes
- 1/2 cup of cooked black beans
- 1/4 cup cherry tomatoes, cut in half
- 2 tablespoons of olive oil
- Juice of 1 lime
- Chopped fresh coriander
- Salt and pepper to taste.

Instructions:

1. In a bowl, mix cooked brown rice with diced avocado, cooked black beans, and halved cherry tomatoes.
2. Dress with olive oil and lime juice.
3. Add chopped fresh cilantro and mix all ingredients well.
4. Season with salt and pepper to taste.
5. Store brown rice and avocado salad in airtight containers and take it to work for a light and tasty lunch.

178. Vegetarian Sandwich with Cream of Avocado

Ingredients for 2 servings:

- 2 whole-grain sandwiches
- 1 ripe avocado, crushed
- 1 carrot, cut into julienne strips
- 1 cucumber, cut into julienne strips
- 1 red bell pepper, cut into strips
- 1/2 cup of soybean sprouts
- 2 tablespoons of vegan mayonnaise
- 1 tablespoon of mustard
- Salt and pepper to taste.

Instructions:

1. Cut the sandwiches in half and spread the avocado cream on both sides.
2. Arrange julienned carrots, julienned cucumbers, bell bell pepper strips, and soybean sprouts on one side of the sandwich.
3. Spread the vegan mayonnaise and mustard on the other side of the sandwich.
4. Close the sandwich and store it in plastic wrap to take to work.

179. Vegan Tabbouleh with Chickpeas.

Ingredients for 2 servings:

- 1 cup cooked whole wheat couscous
- 1/2 cup of cooked chickpeas
- 1/4 cup cherry tomatoes, cut in half
- 1/4 cup cucumber, diced
- 1/4 cup chopped fresh parsley
- 2 tablespoons of olive oil
- Juice of 1 lemon
- Chopped fresh mint
- Salt and pepper to taste.

Instructions:

1. In a bowl, mix cooked whole wheat couscous with cooked chickpeas, halved cherry tomatoes, diced cucumber, and chopped fresh parsley.
2. Season with olive oil and lemon juice.
3. Add chopped fresh mint and mix all ingredients well.
4. Season with salt and pepper to taste.
5. Store the vegan tabbouleh with chickpeas in airtight containers and bring it to work for a light and tasty lunch.

180. Quinoa and Cherry Tomato Salad.

Ingredients for 2 servings:

- 1 cup of cooked quinoa
- 1/2 cup cherry tomatoes, cut in half
- 1/4 cup black olives, pitted and sliced
- 1/4 cup cucumber, diced
- 2 tablespoons of olive oil
- Juice of 1 lemon
- Chopped fresh basil
- Salt and pepper to taste.

Instructions:

1. In a bowl, mix the cooked quinoa with the halved cherry tomatoes, sliced black olives, and diced cucumber.
2. Season with olive oil and lemon juice.
3. Add chopped fresh basil and mix all ingredients well.
4. Season with salt and pepper to taste.
5. Store the quinoa and cherry tomato salad in airtight containers and bring it to work for a light and tasty lunch.

181. Vegan Mushroom and Spinach Sandwich

Ingredients for 2 servings:

- 2 whole-grain vegan sandwiches
- 7 ounces of mushrooms, sliced
- 2 handfuls of fresh spinach
- 2 tablespoons of olive oil
- 1 clove of garlic, minced
- Salt and pepper to taste.
- 2 tablespoons of vegan mayonnaise
- 1 tablespoon of mustard

Instructions:

1. In a skillet, heat olive oil and add fresh spinach. Wilt the spinach until it reduces in volume.
2. Add the mushrooms and minced garlic to the pan and saute until the mushrooms are cooked.
3. Cut the sandwiches in half and spread vegan mayonnaise on both sides.
4. Fill the sandwiches with the mushroom and spinach mixture.
5. Season with salt and pepper to taste.
6. Close the sandwiches and store them in plastic wrap to take to work.

182. Browned Rice Salad with Avocado and Almonds.

Ingredients for 2 servings:

- 1 cup of cooked dehulled rice
- 1 ripe avocado, cut into cubes
- 1/4 cup sliced and roasted almonds
- 2 tablespoons of olive oil
- Juice of 1 lemon
- Chopped fresh parsley
- Salt and pepper to taste.

Instructions:

1. In a bowl, mix cooked dehulled rice with diced avocado and sliced, toasted almonds.
2. Season with olive oil and lemon juice.
3. Add fresh chopped parsley and mix all ingredients well.
4. Season with salt and pepper to taste.
5. Store sbramato rice salad with avocado and almonds in airtight containers and bring it to work for a nutritious and tasty lunch.

183. Cold Spelt with Melon and Mint

Ingredients for 2 servings:

- 1 cup of cooked spelt
- 1 cup diced cantaloupe
- 1/4 cup sliced and roasted almonds
- 2 tablespoons of olive oil
- Juice of 1 lemon
- Chopped fresh mint
- Salt and pepper to taste.

Instructions:

1. In a bowl, mix cooked farro with diced melon and sliced, toasted almonds.
2. Season with olive oil and lemon juice.
3. Add chopped fresh mint and mix all ingredients well.
4. Season with salt and pepper to taste.
5. Store cold farro with melon and mint in airtight containers and take it to work for a light, refreshing lunch.

184. Vegan Sandwich with Hummus and Grilled Peppers.

Ingredients for 2 servings:

- 2 whole-grain vegan sandwiches
- 1/2 cup hummus
- 2 peppers (different colors), cut into strips

- o 2 tablespoons of olive oil
- o Salt and pepper to taste.
- o Arugula

Instructions:

1. Preheat a nonstick grill or frying pan.
2. Brush the bell pepper strips with olive oil and season with salt and pepper.
3. Grill the peppers until tender and slightly charred.
4. Cut the sandwiches in half and spread hummus on both sides.
5. Fill the sandwiches with the grilled bell pepper strips and a few arugula leaves.
6. Close the sandwiches and store them in plastic wrap to take to work.

185. Spelt Salad with Roasted Vegetables.

Ingredients for 2 servings:

- o 1 cup of cooked spelt
- o 1 zucchini, diced
- o 1 eggplant, diced
- o 1 red bell pepper, cut into strips
- o 2 tablespoons of olive oil
- o Salt and pepper to taste.
- o 2 tablespoons balsamic vinegar
- o Chopped fresh parsley

Instructions:

1. Preheat the oven to 200°C (390°F).
2. In a baking dish, distribute the diced zucchini, diced eggplant, and bell pepper strips.
3. Season the vegetables with olive oil, salt and pepper.
4. Roast the vegetables in the oven until soft and lightly browned.
5. In a bowl, mix the cooked farro with the roasted vegetables.
6. Season with balsamic vinegar and fresh chopped parsley.

7. Mix all ingredients well and store the spelt salad with roasted vegetables in airtight containers to take to work.

186. Vegan Tostadas with Avocado Sauce.

Ingredients for 2 servings:

- o 4 vegan tostadas
- o 1 ripe avocado, crushed
- o 1/2 cup cherry tomatoes, cut in half
- o 1/4 cup red onion, thinly sliced
- o 2 tablespoons of olive oil
- o Juice of 1 lime
- o Chopped fresh coriander
- o Salt and pepper to taste.

Instructions:

1. In a bowl, mix mashed avocado with halved cherry tomatoes and thinly sliced red onion.
2. Dress with olive oil and lime juice.
3. Add chopped fresh cilantro and mix all ingredients well.
4. Season with salt and pepper to taste.
5. Spread the avocado mixture over 2 vegan tostadas and top with 2 more tostadas to form a sandwich.
6. Store vegan tostadas with avocado salsa in plastic wrap to take to work.

187. Barley Salad with Tomatoes and Cucumbers.

Ingredients for 2 servings:

- o 1 cup of cooked barley
- o 1/2 cup cherry tomatoes, cut in half
- o 1/2 cup cucumbers, diced
- o 1/4 cup black olives, pitted and sliced
- o 2 tablespoons of olive oil
- o Juice of 1 lemon
- o Chopped fresh parsley
- o Salt and pepper to taste.

Instructions:

1. In a bowl, mix the cooked barley with the halved cherry tomatoes, diced cucumbers, and sliced black olives.
2. Season with olive oil and lemon juice.
3. Add fresh chopped parsley and mix all ingredients well.
4. Season with salt and pepper to taste.
5. Store barley salad with tomatoes and cucumbers in airtight containers and bring it to work for a light and tasty lunch.

188. Vegan Sandwich with Creamed Walnuts and Lettuce

Ingredients for 2 servings:

- 4 slices of whole wheat bread
- 1/2 cup walnuts
- 1 clove of garlic
- 1 tablespoon of lemon juice
- 1 tablespoon apple cider vinegar
- 1 tablespoon of olive oil
- Salt and pepper to taste.
- Lettuce leaves

Instructions:

1. In a blender or food processor, blend the walnuts with the garlic clove, lemon juice, apple cider vinegar, and olive oil until smooth.
2. Season with salt and pepper to taste.
3. Spread the walnut cream on 2 slices of whole wheat bread.
4. Add lettuce leaves on each slice of bread spread with the walnut cream.
5. Close the sandwiches with the other 2 slices of bread and store them in plastic wrap to take to work.

189. Quinoa and Pomegranate Salad.

Ingredients for 2 servings:

- 1 cup of cooked quinoa
- 1/2 cup of pomegranate seeds
- 1/4 cup pecans, toasted and chopped
- 2 tablespoons of olive oil
- Juice of 1 lemon
- Chopped fresh mint
- Salt and pepper to taste.

Instructions:

1. In a bowl, mix the cooked quinoa with the pomegranate seeds and toasted, chopped pecans.
2. Season with olive oil and lemon juice.
3. Add chopped fresh mint and mix all ingredients well.
4. Season with salt and pepper to taste.
5. Store the quinoa and pomegranate salad in airtight containers and take it to work for a light and tasty lunch.

190. Vegan Tacos with Avocado Sauce.

Ingredients for 2 servings:

- 4 corn or whole wheat tortillas
- 1 ripe avocado, crushed
- 1/2 cup cherry tomatoes, cut in half
- 1/4 cup red onion, thinly sliced
- 2 tablespoons of olive oil
- Juice of 1 lime
- Chopped fresh coriander
- Salt and pepper to taste.

Instructions:

1. In a bowl, mix mashed avocado with halved cherry tomatoes and thinly sliced red onion.
2. Dress with olive oil and lime juice.
3. Add chopped fresh cilantro and mix all ingredients well.
4. Season with salt and pepper to taste.

5. Heat tortillas in a frying pan until hot.
6. Fill the tortillas with the avocado salsa and roll them up to form the tacos.
7. Store vegan tacos with avocado salsa in plastic wrap to take to work.

191. Barley and Grilled Zucchini Salad.

Ingredients for 2 servings:

- o 1 cup of cooked barley
- o 1 zucchini, thinly sliced
- o 1/4 cup walnuts, toasted and chopped
- o 2 tablespoons of olive oil
- o Juice of 1 lemon
- o Chopped fresh parsley
- o Salt and pepper to taste.

Instructions:

1. Preheat a nonstick grill or frying pan.
2. Brush the zucchini slices with olive oil and season with salt and pepper.
3. Grill zucchini until tender and slightly charred.
4. In a bowl, mix the cooked barley with the grilled zucchini and toasted and chopped walnuts.
5. Season with lemon juice and fresh chopped parsley.
6. Season with salt and pepper to taste.
7. Store the grilled barley and zucchini salad in airtight containers and bring it to work for a light and tasty lunch.

192. Basmati Rice Salad with Avocado and Chickpeas.

Ingredients for 2 servings:

- o 1 cup of cooked basmati rice
- o 1 ripe avocado, cut into cubes
- o 1/2 cup of cooked chickpeas
- o 1/4 cup cherry tomatoes, cut in half
- o 2 tablespoons of olive oil
- o Juice of 1 lemon
- o Chopped fresh coriander
- o Salt and pepper to taste.

Instructions:

1. In a bowl, mix cooked basmati rice with diced avocado, cooked chickpeas, and halved cherry tomatoes.
2. Season with olive oil and lemon juice.
3. Add chopped fresh cilantro and mix all ingredients well.
4. Season with salt and pepper to taste.
5. Store basmati rice salad with avocado and chickpeas in airtight containers and bring it to work for a light and tasty lunch.

193. Vegan Sandwich with Chickpea Pate and Vegetables.

Ingredients for 2 servings:

- o 2 whole-grain vegan sandwiches
- o 1/2 cup of cooked chickpeas
- o 1 clove of garlic
- o 2 tablespoons tahini
- o 1 tablespoon of lemon juice
- o 1 tablespoon of olive oil
- o Salt and pepper to taste.
- o Grilled peppers
- o Grilled zucchini
- o Grilled eggplant

Instructions:

1. In a blender or food processor, blend the cooked chickpeas with the garlic clove, tahini, lemon juice, and olive oil until smooth.
2. Season with salt and pepper to taste.
3. Cut the sandwiches in half and spread the chickpea pate on both sides.
4. Fill the sandwiches with grilled peppers, grilled zucchini, and grilled eggplant.

5. Close the sandwiches and store them in plastic wrap to take to work.

194. Quinoa and Beet Salad.

Ingredients for 2 servings:

- o 1 cup of cooked quinoa
- o 1 cooked beet, diced
- o 1/4 cup walnuts, toasted and chopped
- o 2 tablespoons of olive oil
- o Juice of 1 orange
- o Chopped fresh parsley
- o Salt and pepper to taste.

Instructions:

1. In a bowl, mix cooked quinoa with diced cooked beet and toasted and chopped walnuts.
2. Season with olive oil and orange juice.
3. Add fresh chopped parsley and mix all ingredients well.
4. Season with salt and pepper to taste.
5. Store the quinoa and beet salad in airtight containers and bring it to work for a light and tasty lunch.

195. Vegan Roll-Ups with Hummus and Vegetables.

Ingredients for 2 servings:

- o 2 whole wheat tortillas or pita bread
- o 1/2 cup hummus
- o 1/4 cup mixed peppers, cut into strips
- o 1/4 cup carrots, cut into julienne strips
- o 1/4 cup cucumber, cut into julienne strips
- o 1/4 cup red onion, thinly sliced
- o Lettuce leaves

Instructions:

1. Roll out whole wheat or pita tortillas on a work surface.

2. Spread the hummus evenly on both tortillas.
3. Arrange the bell pepper strips, julienned carrots, julienned cucumber and red onion slices on the bottom half of each tortilla.
4. Add some lettuce leaves and close the roll-ups by rolling them tightly.
5. Cut each roll-up in half and wrap them in food-grade paper to take to work.

196. Quinoa and Spinach Salad with Almonds.

Ingredients for 2 servings:

- o 1 cup of cooked quinoa
- o 2 handfuls of fresh spinach
- o 1/4 cup sliced and roasted almonds
- o 2 tablespoons of olive oil
- o Juice of 1 lemon
- o Chopped fresh parsley
- o Salt and pepper to taste.

Instructions:

1. In a bowl, mix cooked quinoa with fresh spinach, sliced and toasted almonds.
2. Season with olive oil and lemon juice.
3. Add fresh chopped parsley and mix all ingredients well.
4. Season with salt and pepper to taste.
5. Store the quinoa and spinach salad with almonds in airtight containers and bring it to work for a light and tasty lunch.

197. Vegan Sandwich with Arugula Pesto and Tomatoes.

Ingredients for 2 servings:

- o 2 whole-grain vegan sandwiches
- o 1 cup arugula
- o 1/4 cup of walnuts
- o 1/4 cup of olive oil

- o   1 clove of garlic
- o   Salt and pepper to taste.
- o   Sliced tomatoes

Instructions:

1. In a blender or food processor, blend the arugula with the walnuts, olive oil, and garlic clove until smooth.
2. Season with salt and pepper to taste.
3. Cut the sandwiches in half and spread the arugula pesto on both sides.
4. Fill the sandwiches with tomato slices.
5. Close the sandwiches and store them in plastic wrap to take to work.

198. Couscous Salad with Chickpeas and Vegetables.

Ingredients for 2 servings:

- o   1 cup of cooked couscous
- o   1/2 cup of cooked chickpeas
- o   1/4 cup cherry tomatoes, cut in half
- o   1/4 cup cucumber, diced
- o   1/4 cup mixed peppers, diced
- o   2 tablespoons of olive oil
- o   Juice of 1 lemon
- o   Chopped fresh mint
- o   Salt and pepper to taste.

Instructions:

1. In a bowl, mix the cooked couscous with the cooked chickpeas, halved cherry tomatoes, diced cucumber, and diced mixed peppers.
2. Season with olive oil and lemon juice.
3. Add chopped fresh mint and mix all ingredients well.
4. Season with salt and pepper to taste.
5. Store the couscous salad with chickpeas and vegetables in airtight containers and take it to work for a light and tasty lunch.

199. Grilled Tofu with Vegetables

Ingredients for 2 servings:

- o   1 cup tofu, cut into slices
- o   1 zucchini, thinly sliced
- o   1 eggplant, thinly sliced
- o   1 red bell pepper, cut into strips
- o   2 tablespoons of olive oil
- o   Salt and pepper to taste.
- o   Soy sauce (optional)

Instructions:

1. Preheat a nonstick grill or frying pan.
2. Brush the tofu, zucchini, eggplant, and bell bell pepper slices with olive oil and season with salt and pepper.
3. Grill the tofu and vegetables until tender and slightly charred.
4. If desired, you can marinate the tofu with soy sauce to make it more flavorful.
5. Serve grilled tofu with vegetables as a main dish for your lunch at work.

200. Black Rice Salad with Mango and Avocado

Ingredients for 2 servings:

- o   1 cup of cooked black rice
- o   1 ripe mango, cut into cubes
- o   1 ripe avocado, cut into cubes
- o   2 tablespoons of olive oil
- o   Juice of 1 lime
- o   Chopped fresh coriander
- o   Salt and pepper to taste.

Instructions:

1. In a bowl, mix cooked black rice with diced mango and diced avocado.
2. Dress with olive oil and lime juice.
3. Add chopped fresh cilantro and mix all ingredients well.
4. Season with salt and pepper to taste.

5. Store black rice salad with mango and avocado in airtight containers and take it to work for a light and tasty lunch.

6. With these delicious vegan recipes for lunch at work, you can enjoy nutritious and tasty meals away from home. Enjoy!

CHAPTER 6
60-Day Meal Plan

Introduction

Welcome to our exclusive 60-day meal plan for following an anti-inflammatory diet. This program will help you improve your health by reducing inflammation in the body and providing you with nutritious and tasty meals.

Meal plan guidelines

- Follow a diet rich in fruits and vegetables: Choose seasonal fruits and vegetables that are rich in antioxidants and beneficial nutrients to reduce inflammation.
- Opt for whole grains: Replace refined grains with whole grains such as brown rice, quinoa, spelt and oats, which provide fiber and essential nutrients.
- Include lean protein: Opt for lean protein sources such as legumes, tofu, tempeh, nuts, seeds and oily fish, which help reduce inflammation in the body.
- Use healthy oils: Choose extra virgin olive oil, coconut oil and flaxseed oil, which are rich in omega-3 fatty acids and have anti-inflammatory properties.
- Limit processed foods: Avoid packaged foods high in refined sugars, trans fats and artificial additives, as they can increase inflammation.
- Drink plenty of water: Keep your body hydrated by drinking at least 8 glasses of water a day to promote detoxification and reduce inflammation.

Day 1:

Breakfast - Kiwi and Spinach Smoothie

Snack - Mix of Walnuts and Dried Fruit

Lunch - Quinoa and Avocado Salad

More Snack - Carrots with Beet Hummus

Dinner - Roll-Up of Smoked Salmon and Cream of Avocado

Day 2:

Breakfast - Avocado Toast with Fried Egg

Snack - Fresh Fruit with Yogurt and Mint Sauce

Lunch - Whole wheat pasta with arugula pesto and cherry tomatoes

Other Snack - Pumpkin Hummus

Dinner - Salmon Salad with Avocado and Walnuts

Day 3:

Breakfast - Oatmeal Porridge with Berries

Snack - Banana Coconut Ice Cream

Lunch - Chicken Curry with Vegetables and Brown Rice

More Snack - Vegan Sandwich with Hummus and Grilled Vegetables

Dinner - Quinoa with Broccoli and Walnuts

Day 4:

Breakfast - Banana and Walnut Pancakes

Snack - Oatmeal and Apple Muffins

Lunch - Grilled Salmon with Asparagus and Sweet Potatoes

Other Snack - Antioxidant Green Smoothie

Dinner - Chickpea and Tomato Salad

Day 5:

Breakfast - Almond Butter and Raspberry Jam on Whole Wheat Bread

Snack - Almond and Coconut Bars

Lunch - Chicken and Avocado Wrap

Other Snack - Coconut Mango Smoothie

Dinner - Lemon and Rosemary Chicken with Roasted Potatoes

Day 6:

Breakfast - Omelette with Herbs and Tomatoes

Snack - Grilled Tofu with Peanut and Broccoli Sauce

Lunch - Risotto with Porcini Mushrooms and Spinach

Other Snack - Orange and Ginger Smoothie

Dinner - Quinoa and Bean Burrito with Guacamole

Day 7:

Breakfast - Egg Burrito with Avocado and Tomato Salsa

Snack - Tropical Pineapple and Mango Smoothie

Lunch - Lentil and Vegetable Soup

More Snack - Crispy Baked Chickpeas

Dinner - Tomato and Basil Soup with Crostini

Day 8:

Breakfast - Yogurt, Fruit and Homemade Granola Parfait

Snack - Quinoa Salad with Fresh Vegetables

Lunch - Quinoa and Chickpea Meatballs with Tomato Sauce

Other Snack - Banana and Cocoa Smoothie

Dinner - Salmon and Avocado Salad

Day 9:

Breakfast - Apple Cinnamon Muffins

Snack - Vegan Tostadas with Avocado Sauce

Lunch - Couscous Salad with Grilled Vegetables

More Snack - Energizing Green Smoothie with Kiwi and Spinach

Dinner - Red Lentil Soup with Ginger

Day 10:

Breakfast - Sweet Potato Toast with Avocado Cream

Snack - Basmati Rice Salad with Black Beans

Lunch - Vegan Curry Wrap

Other Snack - Banana and Chocolate Smoothie

Dinner - Chicken Salad with Avocado and Almonds

Day 11:

Breakfast - Whole Wheat Waffles with Fresh Fruit and Maple Syrup

Snack - Melon and Lime Smoothie

Lunch - Spelt Salad with Roasted Vegetables

More Snack - Energizing Smoothie with Mint and Ginger

Dinner - Vegetable Omelette with Spinach and Cherry Tomatoes

Day 12:

Breakfast - Smoothie Bowl with Acai and Coconut

Snack - Quinoa and Spinach Salad with Almonds

Lunch - Cold Spelt with Melon and Mint

Other Snack - Refreshing Cherry Lemon Smoothie

Dinner - Sesame Chicken Bowl with Grilled Vegetables

Day 13:

Breakfast - Scrambled Eggs with Asparagus and Tomatoes

Snack - Vegan Sandwich with Chickpea Pate and Vegetables

Lunch - Vegan Tabbouleh with Chickpeas

Other Snack - Coffee and Cocoa Energy Smoothie

Dinner - Grilled Salmon with Asparagus and Sweet Potatoes

Day 14:

Breakfast - Whole Wheat Banana Bread with Walnuts

Snack - Barley Salad with Tomatoes and Cucumbers

Lunch - Vegan Sandwich with Creamed Walnuts and Lettuce

More Snack - Refreshing Smoothie with Mint and Lime

Dinner - Chicken with Sun-Dried Tomatoes and Spinach

Day 15:

Breakfast - Buckwheat Crepes with Berries

Snack - Lavender and Honey Zen Smoothie

Lunch - Brown Rice and Avocado Salad

Other Snack - Energizing Orange and Carrot Smoothie

Dinner - Chickpea and Arugula Salad

Day 16:

Breakfast - Anti-Inflammatory Green Smoothie

Snack - Spelt and Cucumber Salad

Lunch - Vegetarian Sandwich with Cream of Avocado

More Snack - Raspberry Vanilla Smoothie

Dinner - Chicken Curry with Vegetables

Day 17:

Breakfast - Zucchini and Peppers Omelette

Snack - Quinoa and Beet Salad

Lunch - Grilled Tofu with Sautéed Vegetables

More Snack - Energizing Green Tea and Ginger Smoothie

Dinner - Grilled Shrimp with Mango and Avocado Sauce

Day 18:

Breakfast - Quinoa Porridge with Dried Fruit

Snack - Spelt Salad with Roasted Vegetables

Lunch - Watermelon and Strawberry Smoothie

Other Snack - Tonifying Smoothie with Pomegranate and Orange

Dinner - Vegetable Omelette with Smoked Salmon

Day 19:

Breakfast - Pumpkin Pancakes with Chia Seeds

Snack - Basmati Rice Salad with Almonds and Raisins

Lunch - Couscous with Chickpeas and Vegetables

More Snack - Celery and Cucumber Detox Smoothie

Dinner - Sesame Chicken Bowl with Grilled Vegetables

Day 20:

Breakfast - Coconut and Pineapple Smoothie

Snack - Quinoa and Avocado Salad with Black Beans

Lunch - Quinoa Salad with Cucumbers and Tomatoes

More Snack - Goji Berry and Blueberry Antioxidant Smoothie

Dinner - Grilled Salmon with Asparagus and Sweet Potatoes

Day 21:

Breakfast - Coffee and Banana Smoothie

Snack - Energizing Smoothie with Mint and Ginger

Lunch - Lentil and Avocado Salad

Other Snack - Mango and Coconut Smoothie

Dinner - Risotto with Porcini Mushrooms and Spinach

Day 22:

Breakfast - Avocado Toast with Fried Egg

Snack - Banana and Cocoa Smoothie

Lunch - Chicken Curry with Vegetables and Brown Rice

Other Snack - Refreshing Cherry Lemon Smoothie

Dinner - Chicken Salad with Avocado and Almonds

Day 23:

Breakfast - Kiwi and Spinach Smoothie

Snack - Green Tea Ginger Energy Smoothie

Lunch - Grilled Shrimp with Mango and Avocado Sauce

More Snack - Energizing Coffee and Cocoa Smoothie

Dinner - Chicken with Mango Sauce and Basmati Rice

Day 24:

Breakfast - Oatmeal Porridge with Berries

Snack - Barley and Chickpea Salad

Lunch - Quinoa and Avocado Salad with Black Beans

More Snack - Energizing Smoothie with Mint and Ginger

Dinner - Lemon and Rosemary Chicken with Roasted Potatoes

Day 25:

Breakfast - Anti-Inflammatory Green Smoothie

Snack - Melon and Lime Smoothie

Lunch - Spelt Salad with Roasted Vegetables

Other Snack - Tonifying Smoothie with Pomegranate and Orange

Dinner - Vegetable Omelette with Spinach and Cherry Tomatoes

Day 26:

Breakfast - Pumpkin Pancakes with Chia Seeds

Snack - Quinoa and Beet Salad

Lunch - Grilled Tofu with Sautéed Vegetables

More Snack - Energizing Smoothie with Green Tea and Ginger

Dinner - Grilled Shrimp with Mango and Avocado Sauce

Day 27:

Breakfast - Zucchini and Peppers Omelette

Snack - Quinoa and Avocado Salad with Black Beans

Lunch - Quinoa Salad with Cucumbers and Tomatoes

More Snack - Celery and Cucumber Detox Smoothie

Dinner - Grilled Salmon with Asparagus and Sweet Potatoes

Day 28:

Breakfast - Coconut and Pineapple Smoothie

Snack - Spelt Salad with Roasted Vegetables

Lunch - Watermelon and Strawberry Smoothie

Other Snack - Tonifying Smoothie with Pomegranate and Orange

Dinner - Vegetable Omelette with Smoked Salmon

Day 29:

Breakfast - Banana and Walnut Pancakes

Snack - Basmati Rice Salad with Almonds and Raisins

Lunch - Couscous with Chickpeas and Vegetables

More Snack - Celery and Cucumber Detox Smoothie

Dinner - Sesame Chicken Bowl with Grilled Vegetables

Day 30:

Breakfast - Smoothie Bowl with Acai and Coconut

Snack - Energizing Smoothie with Mint and Ginger

Lunch - Lentil and Avocado Salad

Other Snack - Mango and Coconut Smoothie

Dinner - Risotto with Porcini Mushrooms and Spinach

Day 31:

Breakfast - Avocado Toast with Fried Egg

Snack - Banana and Cocoa Smoothie

Lunch - Chicken Curry with Vegetables and Brown Rice

Other Snack - Refreshing Cherry Lemon Smoothie

Dinner - Chicken Salad with Avocado and Almonds

Day 32:

Breakfast - Kiwi and Spinach Smoothie

Snack - Green Tea Ginger Energy Smoothie

Lunch - Grilled Shrimp with Mango and Avocado Sauce

More Snack - Energizing Coffee and Cocoa Smoothie

Dinner - Chicken with Mango Sauce and Basmati Rice

Day 33:

Breakfast - Oatmeal Porridge with Berries

Snack - Barley and Chickpea Salad

Lunch - Quinoa and Avocado Salad with Black Beans

More Snack - Energizing Smoothie with Mint and Ginger

Dinner - Lemon and Rosemary Chicken with Roasted Potatoes

Day 34:

Breakfast - Anti-Inflammatory Green Smoothie

Snack - Melon and Lime Smoothie

Lunch - Spelt Salad with Roasted Vegetables

Other Snack - Tonifying Smoothie with Pomegranate and Orange

Dinner - Vegetable Omelette with Spinach and Cherry Tomatoes

Day 35:

Breakfast - Pumpkin Pancakes with Chia Seeds

Snack - Quinoa and Beet Salad

Lunch - Grilled Tofu with Sautéed Vegetables

More Snack - Energizing Smoothie with Green Tea and Ginger

Dinner - Grilled Shrimp with Mango and Avocado Sauce

Day 36:

Breakfast - Zucchini and Peppers Omelette

Snack - Quinoa and Avocado Salad with Black Beans

Lunch - Quinoa Salad with Cucumbers and Tomatoes

More Snack - Celery and Cucumber Detox Smoothie

Dinner - Grilled Salmon with Asparagus and Sweet Potatoes

Day 37:

Breakfast - Coconut and Pineapple Smoothie

Snack - Spelt Salad with Roasted Vegetables

Lunch - Watermelon and Strawberry Smoothie

Other Snack - Tonifying Smoothie with Pomegranate and Orange

Dinner - Vegetable Omelette with Smoked Salmon

Day 38:

Breakfast - Smoothie Bowl with Acai and Coconut

Snack - Energizing Smoothie with Mint and Ginger

Lunch - Lentil and Avocado Salad

Other Snack - Mango and Coconut Smoothie

Dinner - Risotto with Porcini Mushrooms and Spinach

Day 39:

Breakfast - Avocado Toast with Fried Egg

Snack - Banana and Cocoa Smoothie

Lunch - Chicken Curry with Vegetables and Brown Rice

Other Snack - Refreshing Cherry Lemon Smoothie

Dinner - Chicken Salad with Avocado and Almonds

Day 40:

Breakfast - Kiwi and Spinach Smoothie

Snack - Green Tea Ginger Energy Smoothie

Lunch - Grilled Shrimp with Mango and Avocado Sauce

More Snack - Energizing Coffee and Cocoa Smoothie

Dinner - Chicken with Mango Sauce and Basmati Rice

Day 41:

Breakfast - Oatmeal Porridge with Berries

Snack - Barley and Chickpea Salad

Lunch - Quinoa and Avocado Salad with Black Beans

More Snack - Energizing Smoothie with Mint and Ginger

Dinner - Lemon and Rosemary Chicken with Roasted Potatoes

Day 42:

Breakfast - Anti-Inflammatory Green Smoothie

Snack - Melon and Lime Smoothie

Lunch - Spelt Salad with Roasted Vegetables

Other Snack - Tonifying Smoothie with Pomegranate and Orange

Dinner - Vegetable Omelette with Spinach and Cherry Tomatoes

Day 43:

Breakfast - Pumpkin Pancakes with Chia Seeds

Snack - Quinoa and Beet Salad

Lunch - Grilled Tofu with Sautéed Vegetables

More Snack - Energizing Green Tea and Ginger Smoothie

Dinner - Grilled Shrimp with Mango and Avocado Sauce

Day 44:

Breakfast - Zucchini and Peppers Omelette

Snack - Quinoa and Avocado Salad with Black Beans

Lunch - Quinoa Salad with Cucumbers and Tomatoes

More Snack - Celery and Cucumber Detox Smoothie

Dinner - Grilled Salmon with Asparagus and Sweet Potatoes

Day 45:

Breakfast - Coconut and Pineapple Smoothie

Snack - Spelt Salad with Roasted Vegetables

Lunch - Watermelon and Strawberry Smoothie

Other Snack - Tonifying Smoothie with Pomegranate and Orange

Dinner - Vegetable Omelette with Smoked Salmon

Day 46:

Breakfast - Smoothie Bowl with Acai and Coconut

Snack - Energizing Smoothie with Mint and Ginger

Lunch - Lentil and Avocado Salad

Other Snack - Mango and Coconut Smoothie

Dinner - Risotto with Porcini Mushrooms and Spinach

Day 47:

Breakfast - Avocado Toast with Fried Egg

Snack - Banana and Cocoa Smoothie

Lunch - Chicken Curry with Vegetables and Brown Rice

Other Snack - Refreshing Cherry Lemon Smoothie

Dinner - Chicken Salad with Avocado and Almonds

Day 48:

Breakfast - Kiwi and Spinach Smoothie

Snack - Green Tea Ginger Energy Smoothie

Lunch - Grilled Shrimp with Mango and Avocado Sauce

More Snack - Energizing Coffee and Cocoa Smoothie

Dinner - Chicken with Mango Sauce and Basmati Rice

Day 49:

Breakfast - Oatmeal Porridge with Berries

Snack - Barley and Chickpea Salad

Lunch - Quinoa and Avocado Salad with Black Beans

More Snack - Energizing Smoothie with Mint and Ginger

Dinner - Lemon and Rosemary Chicken with Roasted Potatoes

Day 50:

Breakfast - Anti-Inflammatory Green Smoothie

Snack - Melon and Lime Smoothie

Lunch - Spelt Salad with Roasted Vegetables

Other Snack - Tonifying Smoothie with Pomegranate and Orange

Dinner - Vegetable Omelette with Spinach and Cherry Tomatoes

Day 51:

Breakfast - Pumpkin Pancakes with Chia Seeds

Snack - Quinoa and Beet Salad

Lunch - Grilled Tofu with Sautéed Vegetables

More Snack - Energizing Green Tea and Ginger Smoothie

Dinner - Grilled Shrimp with Mango and Avocado Sauce

Day 52:

Breakfast - Zucchini and Peppers Omelette

Snack - Quinoa and Avocado Salad with Black Beans

Lunch - Quinoa Salad with Cucumbers and Tomatoes

More Snack - Celery and Cucumber Detox Smoothie

Dinner - Grilled Salmon with Asparagus and Sweet Potatoes

Day 53:

Breakfast - Coconut and Pineapple Smoothie

Snack - Spelt Salad with Roasted Vegetables

Lunch - Watermelon and Strawberry Smoothie

Other Snack - Tonifying Smoothie with Pomegranate and Orange

Dinner - Vegetable Omelette with Smoked Salmon

Day 54:

Breakfast - Smoothie Bowl with Acai and Coconut

Snack - Energizing Smoothie with Mint and Ginger

Lunch - Lentil and Avocado Salad

Other Snack - Mango and Coconut Smoothie

Dinner - Risotto with Porcini Mushrooms and Spinach

Day 55:

Breakfast - Avocado Toast with Fried Egg

Snack - Banana and Cocoa Smoothie

Lunch - Chicken Curry with Vegetables and Brown Rice

Other Snack - Refreshing Cherry Lemon Smoothie

Dinner - Chicken Salad with Avocado and Almonds

Day 56:

Breakfast - Kiwi and Spinach Smoothie

Snack - Green Tea Ginger Energy Smoothie

Lunch - Grilled Shrimp with Mango and Avocado Sauce

More Snack - Energizing Coffee and Cocoa Smoothie

Dinner - Chicken with Mango Sauce and Basmati Rice

Day 57:

Breakfast - Oatmeal Porridge with Berries

Snack - Barley and Chickpea Salad

Lunch - Quinoa and Avocado Salad with Black Beans

More Snack - Energizing Smoothie with Mint and Ginger

Dinner - Lemon and Rosemary Chicken with Roasted Potatoes

Day 58:

Breakfast - Anti-Inflammatory Green Smoothie

Snack - Melon and Lime Smoothie

Lunch - Spelt Salad with Roasted Vegetables

Other Snack - Tonifying Smoothie with Pomegranate and Orange

Dinner - Vegetable Omelette with Spinach and Cherry Tomatoes

Day 59:

Breakfast - Pumpkin Pancakes with Chia Seeds

Snack - Quinoa and Beet Salad

Lunch - Grilled Tofu with Sautéed Vegetables

More Snack - Energizing Green Tea and Ginger Smoothie

Dinner - Grilled Shrimp with Mango and Avocado Sauce

Day 60:

Breakfast - Zucchini and Peppers Omelette

Snack - Quinoa and Avocado Salad with Black Beans

Lunch - Quinoa Salad with Cucumbers and Tomatoes

More Snack - Celery and Cucumber Detox Smoothie

Dinner - Grilled Salmon with Asparagus and Sweet Potatoes

Bonus 1: Accessible Physical Activity Program to Support Anti-Inflammatory Effect.

Introduction

Welcome to Bonus 1 of our cookbook. In this bonus, we will provide you with a physical activity program accessible to everyone, designed to support the anti-inflammatory effect of the diet. The proposed exercises are simple, suitable for beginners, and can be performed at home without the need for special equipment.

Day 1 - Energizing Walk

Duration: 30 minutes

Description: Start your program with an energy walk outdoors or on the treadmill. Walk at a comfortable pace, focusing on breathing and enjoying your surroundings. Walking is an excellent cardiovascular exercise that helps stimulate the circulatory system and reduce inflammation.

Day 2 - Strength Exercises at Body Weight

Duration: 20 minutes

Description: Perform strength exercises using only your body weight, without the need for equipment. For example, leg squats (squats) help strengthen leg and gluteal muscles. Arm push-ups (push-ups) work the chest, arms and shoulders. Planks engage the abs and help stabilize the core. Squats and push-ups on the arms are performed in 3 sets of 10 repetitions each, while the plank is held for 30 seconds in 3 sets.

Day 3 - Stretching for Flexibility

Duration: 15 minutes

Description: Devote yourself to a short stretching session to improve flexibility and reduce muscle tension. Lie on the floor and stretch the main muscles, such as the muscles in your legs, arms and back. Hold each position for 15-30 seconds and repeat 2-3 times.

Day 4 - Active Rest

Description: Today is the day for active rest. Do light stretching or a relaxing walk to promote muscle recovery.

Day 5 - Cardiovascular Interval Training

Duration: 25 minutes

Description: Choose a cardiovascular exercise you enjoy, such as skipping, jumping jacks or mountain climbers. Perform the activity in intervals, alternating moments of intense exertion with moments of active recovery. For example, skipping for 30 seconds at full speed, followed by 30 seconds of light walking or active recovery. Repeat the alternation for 25 minutes.

Day 6 - Stability and Balance Exercises

Duration: 15 minutes

Description: Focus on exercises that improve stability and balance, such as side lunges, leg raises and bicycle crunches. Side lunges are performed in 2 sets of 10 repetitions for each leg. Leg raises are performed in 3 sets of 15 repetitions for each leg. Bicycle sit-ups are performed in 3 sets of 20 repetitions.

Day 7 - Active Rest

Description: Enjoy another day of active rest with a relaxing walk or some deep breathing exercises.

Day 8 - Training with The Shots

Duration: 15 minutes

Description: Do running sprints in short intervals, followed by short recovery breaks. These sprints help boost metabolism and improve cardiovascular fitness. Perform 5 running sprints of 30 seconds each, followed by 30 seconds of light walking.

Day 9 - Breathing and Relaxation

Duration: 10 minutes

Description: Devote yourself to a short session of deep breathing and relaxation exercises to reduce stress and promote overall well-being. Sit in a comfortable position, close your eyes and breathe deeply, filling your lungs completely. Exhale slowly and deeply. Repeat for 5 to 10 minutes.

Day 10 - Exercises for Mobility

Duration: 15 minutes

Description: Conclude your program with exercises to improve joint mobility and promote better posture. Do shoulder rotations, knee bends and neck rotations, keeping each movement fluid and controlled.

Conclusions

This exercise program is designed to be accessible to everyone, without the need for an instructor or expensive equipment. These are simple but effective exercises that you can easily perform at home to support the anti-inflammatory effect of your diet. Remember to consult your doctor before starting any exercise program, and tailor it to your abilities and preferences. Stay consistent and enjoy the benefits that physical activity can bring to your life. Enjoy your workout!

Bonus 2: Stress Management Guide for an Anti-Inflammatory Life

Introduction

Stress can have a significant impact on overall health and well-being. Proper stress management is essential to support the anti-inflammatory effect of diet and maintain balance in body and mind. In this bonus, we will provide practical strategies for managing stress and promoting anti-inflammatory living.

Strategy 1: Breath Awareness

One of the simplest and most effective techniques for managing stress is breath awareness. Deep, mindful breathing helps calm the nervous system, reduce muscle tension and promote a state of calm and relaxation.

Conscious Breathing Exercise:

- Sit in a comfortable position with your back straight and shoulders relaxed.
- Close your eyes and place one hand on your chest and the other on your abdomen.
- Start breathing deeply and slowly through your nose, feeling your chest and abdomen expand.
- Exhale slowly through your mouth, feeling your chest and abdomen contract.
- Keep breathing this way for a few minutes, focusing only on your breathing and trying to push thoughts and worries away.

Strategy 2: Progressive Muscle Relaxation

Progressive muscle relaxation is an effective technique to relax the body and get rid of physical tension caused by stress.

Progressive Muscle Relaxation Exercise:

- Lie down or sit in a comfortable position.
- Focus on one muscle group at a time, such as the shoulders or legs.
- Voluntarily contract the muscles of the selected group for 5-10 seconds.
- Release the tension and let go of the contraction, feeling the muscles become soft and relaxed.
- Move on to another muscle group and repeat the process, proceeding gradually throughout the body.

Strategy 3: Relaxation Activities

Making time for yourself and engaging in relaxing activities can help reduce stress and promote well-being.

Some relaxation activities to try include:

- Reading a book or listening to relaxing music
- Taking a nature walk
- Do yoga or practice meditation
- Taking a hot shower or a relaxing bath

Strategy 4: Maintaining a Routine

Maintaining a regular routine can help reduce stress and promote anti-inflammatory living. Organize your days in a structured way, including time for sleep, healthy eating, physical activity and relaxation.

Strategy 5: Social Support

Social support is crucial for stress management. Talk to friends, family members or seek out a support group where you can share your experiences and receive emotional support.

Conclusions

Stress management is a key element of anti-inflammatory living. Use these stress management strategies in your daily routine to reduce inflammation levels in your body and improve your overall well-being. Remember that each individual is unique, so find the strategies that best suit you and your situation.

Bonus 3: 7-Day Anti-Inflammatory Detox Program

Introduction

The 7-day anti-inflammatory detox program is an effective way to cleanse the body of accumulated toxins and reduce inflammation. This program is based on a diet rich in anti-inflammatory foods and nutrients, which help support immune system function and improve overall health.

Day 1: Breakfast - Smoothie Detox

All the ingredients are intended for 2 persons:

- o 1 cup of fresh spinach
- o 1 ripe banana
- o 1 cup of fresh or frozen pineapple
- o 1/2 cup of Greek yogurt
- o 1 cup of sugar-free almond milk

Blend all ingredients until smooth and homogeneous. Serve chilled.

Day 1: Lunch - Quinoa Salad and Vegetables

All the ingredients are intended for 2 persons:

- o 1 cup of cooked quinoa
- o 1/2 cucumber, diced
- o 1 red bell pepper, diced
- o 1 carrot, grated
- o 1/4 cup fresh parsley, chopped
- o 2 tablespoons of olive oil
- o Juice of 1 lemon
- o Salt and pepper to taste.

Mix all ingredients in a large bowl and season with olive oil, lemon juice, salt and pepper.

Day 1: Dinner - Baked Salmon with Asparagus

All the ingredients are intended for 2 persons:

- o 2 salmon fillets
- o 1 bunch of fresh asparagus
- o 2 tablespoons of olive oil
- o Juice of 1 lemon
- o 2 cloves of garlic, minced
- o Salt and pepper to taste.

Preparation:

1. Preheat the oven to 400°F (200°C).
2. Arrange the salmon fillets and asparagus on a baking sheet.
3. Season with olive oil, lemon juice, minced garlic, salt and pepper.
4. Bake for about 15-20 minutes or until salmon is cooked and vegetables are tender.

Day 2: Breakfast - Oats with Fresh Fruit

All the ingredients are intended for 2 persons:

- o 1 cup of oatmeal
- o 1 cup unsweetened coconut milk
- o 1/2 cup fresh strawberries, cut into pieces
- o 1/2 banana, sliced
- o 1 tablespoon of chia seeds
- o 1 tablespoon chopped walnuts

Preparation:

1. In a saucepan, bring oatmeal to a boil with coconut milk.
2. Reduce the heat and simmer for about 5 minutes or until the oats are soft and creamy.
3. Transfer the oats to a bowl and add the strawberries, banana, chia seeds, and chopped nuts. Mix well and serve warm.

Day 2: Lunch - Chicken and Avocado Salad

All the ingredients are intended for 2 persons:

- o 2 cups cooked chicken breast, diced
- o 1 ripe avocado, cut into cubes
- o 1/2 cup cherry tomatoes, cut in half
- o 1/4 cup red onion, thinly sliced
- o 2 tablespoons of olive oil
- o Juice of 1 lime
- o 1 tablespoon fresh cilantro, chopped
- o Salt and pepper to taste.

Preparation:

1. In a large bowl, mix the chicken, avocado, cherry tomatoes, and onion.
2. Season with olive oil, lime juice, fresh cilantro, salt and pepper. Stir well to blend flavors.

Day 2: Dinner - Fish Tacos

All the ingredients are intended for 2 persons:

- o 2 white fish fillets (e.g., cod or sea bass)
- o 1 tablespoon of olive oil
- o 1 tablespoon paprika
- o 1 teaspoon cumin
- o 1/2 teaspoon garlic powder
- o 1/2 teaspoon chili powder
- o Salt and pepper to taste.
- o Lime juice drops
- o 4 corn tortillas

Preparation:

1. In a bowl, mix olive oil, paprika, cumin, garlic powder, chili powder, salt and pepper.
2. Brush the fish with the seasoning mixture and add a few drops of lime juice.
3. Heat a nonstick skillet over medium-high heat and cook the fish for 3-4 minutes on each side, until cooked through and flaking easily with a fork.

4. Reheat tortillas and stuff with fish and other vegetables to taste. Fold the tortillas in half and serve.

Day 3: Breakfast - Detox Green Smoothie

All the ingredients are intended for 2 persons:

- o 1 cup of fresh spinach
- o 1 green apple, peeled and cut into pieces
- o 1/2 cucumber, diced
- o 1/2 ripe avocado
- o 1 cup of coconut water

Blend all ingredients until smooth and homogeneous. Serve chilled.

Day 3: Lunch - Lentil and Vegetable Salad

All the ingredients are intended for 2 persons:

- o 1 cup of cooked lentils
- o 1/2 cup yellow peppers, diced
- o 1/2 cup cherry tomatoes, cut in half
- o 1/4 cup red onion, thinly sliced
- o 2 tablespoons of olive oil
- o Juice of 1 lemon
- o 1 teaspoon dried oregano
- o Salt and pepper to taste.

Mix all ingredients in a large bowl and season with olive oil, lemon juice, dried oregano, salt and pepper.

Day 3: Dinner - Vegetable and Quinoa Soup

All the ingredients are intended for 2 persons:

- o 1 cup of cooked quinoa
- o 2 cups of vegetable broth
- o 1 zucchini, diced
- o 1 carrot, cut into thin rounds
- o 1 celery stalk, cut into slices
- o 1/2 cup of cooked black beans
- o 1 teaspoon turmeric powder
- o 1/2 teaspoon black pepper
- o Salt to taste.

Preparation:

1. In a pot, bring vegetable broth to a boil.
2. Add the quinoa, vegetables, and beans.
3. Season with turmeric, black pepper and salt. Cook over medium-low heat for about 15 minutes or until vegetables are tender and quinoa is cooked.
4. Serve hot.

Day 4: Breakfast - Oat and Banana Pancakes

All the ingredients are intended for 2 persons:

- o 1 cup of oatmeal
- o 1 ripe banana
- o 2 eggs
- o 1 teaspoon cinnamon powder
- o 1/2 teaspoon baking powder
- o Coconut oil to grease the pan

Preparation:

1. In a bowl, mash the banana with a fork until pureed.
2. Add the oatmeal, eggs, cinnamon and baking powder. Mix well until a smooth dough is obtained.
3. Heat a nonstick skillet over medium-low heat and grease with coconut oil.
4. Pour a ladleful of batter into the pan and cook for a few minutes on each side, until the pancakes are golden brown and cooked through.

Day 4: Lunch - Chicken and Avocado Wrap

All the ingredients are intended for 2 persons:

- o 2 whole wheat tortillas
- o 1 cooked chicken breast, cut into strips
- o 1 ripe avocado, cut into slices
- o 1 cup of shredded lettuce
- o 1/4 cup cherry tomatoes, cut in half
- o 2 tablespoons light mayonnaise
- o Juice of 1 lime
- o Salt and pepper to taste.

Preparation:

1. Heat the tortillas slightly in a skillet or in the microwave to make them softer and more pliable.
2. Spread mayonnaise on the tortillas.
3. Add the chicken, avocado, lettuce, and cherry tomatoes.
4. Season with lime juice, salt and pepper.
5. Roll the tortillas and serve.

Day 4: Dinner - Steamed Fish with Vegetables

All the ingredients are intended for 2 persons:

- o 2 white fish fillets (e.g., cod or sea bass)
- o 1 zucchini, thinly sliced
- o 1 carrot, cut into sticks
- o 1 tablespoon of olive oil
- o Juice of 1 lemon
- o 1/2 teaspoon dried thyme
- o Salt and pepper to taste.

Preparation:

1. Prepare a steamer basket and bring water to a boil.
2. Season the fish fillets with olive oil, lemon juice, thyme, salt and pepper.
3. Arrange the vegetables in the bottom of the steamer basket and place the fish fillets on top of the vegetables.
4. Cover and steam for about 10-15 minutes or until the fish is cooked.
5. Serve hot.

Day 5: Breakfast - Antioxidant Smoothie

All the ingredients are intended for 2 persons:

- o 1 cup of fresh or frozen blueberries
- o 1 ripe banana
- o 1/2 cup of Greek yogurt
- o 1/2 cup of almond milk
- o 1 tablespoon of chia seeds
- o 1 teaspoon of honey (optional)

Blend all ingredients until smooth and homogeneous. Add honey if more sweetness is desired. Serve chilled.

Day 5: Lunch - Quinoa, Chickpea and Vegetable Salad

All the ingredients are intended for 2 persons:

- o 1 cup of cooked quinoa
- o 1 cup of cooked chickpeas
- o 1/2 cup red peppers, diced
- o 1/2 cup cucumbers, diced
- o 1/4 cup red onion, thinly sliced
- o 2 tablespoons of olive oil
- o Juice of 1 lemon
- o 1 teaspoon dried oregano
- o Salt and pepper to taste.

Mix all ingredients in a large bowl and season with olive oil, lemon juice, dried oregano, salt and pepper.

Day 5: Dinner - Baked Salmon with Asparagus

All the ingredients are intended for 2 persons:

- o 2 salmon fillets
- o 1 bunch of asparagus, washed and stripped of the woody part
- o 2 tablespoons of olive oil
- o Juice of 1 lemon
- o 2 cloves of garlic, finely chopped
- o 1 teaspoon paprika
- o Salt and pepper to taste.

Preparation:

1. Preheat the oven to 200°C (390°F).
2. Arrange the salmon fillets and asparagus on a baking sheet lined with baking paper.
3. Season with olive oil, lemon juice, minced garlic, paprika, salt and pepper.
4. Bake for about 15-20 minutes or until salmon is cooked and asparagus is tender.

Day 6: Breakfast - Banana and Zucchini Pancakes

All the ingredients are intended for 2 persons:

- o 1 ripe banana
- o 1 zucchini, finely grated
- o 2 eggs
- o 1/2 cup oatmeal
- o 1 teaspoon cinnamon powder
- o 1/2 teaspoon baking powder
- o Coconut oil to grease the pan

Preparation:

1. In a bowl, mash the banana with a fork until pureed.
2. Add the grated zucchini, eggs, oatmeal, cinnamon, and baking powder. Mix well until the mixture is smooth.
3. Heat a nonstick skillet over medium-low heat and grease with coconut oil.
4. Pour a ladleful of batter into the pan and cook for a few minutes on each side, until the pancakes are golden brown and cooked through.

Day 6: Lunch - Chicken and Avocado Salad

All the ingredients are intended for 2 persons:

- o 2 cups of cooked, diced chicken
- o 1 ripe avocado, cut into slices
- o 1 cup cherry tomatoes, cut in half
- o 1/4 cup red onion, thinly sliced
- o 2 tablespoons of olive oil
- o Juice of 1 lime
- o 1 teaspoon paprika
- o Salt and pepper to taste.

Preparation:

1. In a large bowl, combine the chicken, avocado, cherry tomatoes, and red onion.
2. Season with olive oil, lime juice, paprika, salt and pepper. Mix well to blend flavors.
3. Serve cold.

Day 6: Dinner - Potato and Broccoli Soup

All the ingredients are intended for 2 persons:

- o 2 medium potatoes, diced
- o 2 cups broccoli, cut into small pieces
- o 1 onion, finely chopped
- o 2 cloves of garlic, finely chopped
- o 4 cups of vegetable broth
- o 1/2 cup of almond milk
- o 1 teaspoon turmeric powder
- o Salt and pepper to taste.

Preparation:

1. In a large pot, heat some olive oil and add the onion and garlic. Brown until they become translucent.
2. Add the potatoes and broccoli and cook for a few minutes.
3. Pour in vegetable broth and bring to a boil. Reduce heat and cook over medium heat until potatoes and broccoli are tender.
4. Add the almond milk and turmeric and mix well. Cook for another 5 minutes.
5. Blend the soup with an immersion blender until smooth and creamy. Adjust for salt and pepper.
6. Serve hot.

Day 7: Breakfast - Detox Green Smoothie

All the ingredients are intended for 2 persons:

- o 1 cup of fresh spinach
- o 1 kiwi, peeled and cut into pieces
- o 1/2 ripe avocado
- o 1/2 cup fresh or frozen pineapple
- o 1 cup of coconut milk
- o 1 tablespoon of chia seeds

Blend all ingredients until smooth and homogeneous. Add water or coconut milk to reach desired consistency. Serve chilled.

Day 7: Lunch - Quinoa Salad with Grilled Vegetables

All the ingredients are intended for 2 persons:

- o 1 cup of cooked quinoa
- o 1 zucchini, thinly sliced
- o 1 red bell pepper, thinly sliced
- o 1 red onion, thinly sliced
- o 1 tablespoon of olive oil
- o Juice of 1 lemon
- o 2 tablespoons fresh parsley, finely chopped
- o Salt and pepper to taste.

Preparation:

1. In a bowl, mix zucchini, bell bell pepper, and onion slices with olive oil, lemon juice, salt, and pepper.
2. Grill vegetables on a hot grill until slightly charred and keep aside.
3. In a large bowl, combine the cooked quinoa with the grilled vegetables and chopped parsley.
4. Season with a drizzle of olive oil and serve at room temperature.

Day 7: Dinner - Grilled Salmon with Avocado Salad

All the ingredients are intended for 2 persons:

- o 2 salmon fillets
- o Juice of 1 lemon
- o 2 tablespoons of olive oil
- o Salt and pepper to taste.
- o 1 ripe avocado, cut into slices
- o 2 cups of mixed salad
- o 1/4 cup cherry tomatoes, cut in half
- o 1/4 cup cucumbers, cut into slices
- o 2 tablespoons apple cider vinegar

Preparation:

1. In a bowl, marinate the salmon fillets with lemon juice, olive oil, salt and pepper for about 30 minutes.
2. Heat a grill and cook the salmon for a few minutes on each side until cooked.
3. In a large bowl, mix salad mix with avocado slices, cherry tomatoes, and cucumbers. Season with apple cider vinegar.
4. Serve the grilled salmon on the bed of avocado salad.

With this we complete the 7-day anti-inflammatory detox program. Each recipe has been selected to provide maximum anti-inflammatory support while providing a wide variety of flavors and nutrients beneficial to the body. It is recommended to follow this program only if there are no special health conditions or dietary restrictions. Before embarking on any significant changes in diet or physical activity, it is recommended that you consult a health care professional. Enjoy your journey to a healthier, more sustainable body!

Conclusion

Congratulations! If you have made it this far, it means you have completed an exciting journey toward discovering the anti-inflammatory power of diet. This cookbook was created with love and dedication to provide you with a practical and tasty guide to a healthier, more balanced lifestyle.

Together we explored the process of inflammation in the body and how diet can play a key role in managing and reducing it. We discovered a wide range of foods, herbs, spices and seasonings that can help you fight inflammation and promote your health naturally.

The recipes offered have been carefully selected to be delicious, nutritious and anti-inflammatory. Each dish is designed to be prepared with ease, saving valuable time in your kitchen and allowing you to fully enjoy food without guilt.

But the journey to anti-inflammatory living doesn't stop there! In our cookbook, you'll also find three special bonuses: a physical activity program to support the anti-inflammatory effect of the diet, a stress management guide to promote mental balance, and a 7-day detox program to start cleansing your body of impurities and toxins.

Remember, change does not happen overnight, but with small, steady, conscious steps. We are here to support you every step of the way on your path to a healthier life in harmony with yourself.

Thank you for choosing our cookbook and allowing us to be part of your journey to health. Whether you are a beginner or an expert in the world of anti-inflammatory cooking, we hope these recipes will inspire you to experiment with new flavors, take care of your body, and live each day with joy and vitality.

Bon appetite and good health!

Martha Johnson

Made in United States
Orlando, FL
16 September 2023

36991452R00061